START RIGHT!

The Definitive Guide to
Joining a Gym for the First Time

by Gino A. Spada

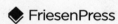

FriesenPress

Suite 300 - 990 Fort St
Victoria, BC, V8V 3K2
Canada

www.friesenpress.com

ISBN
978-1-5255-9118-1 (Hardcover)
978-1-5255-9117-4 (Paperback)
978-1-5255-9119-8 (eBook)

1. Health & Fitness, Exercise

Distributed to the trade by The Ingram Book Company

TABLE OF CONTENTS

DEDICATION

I would like to dedicate this book to all of the past, present, and even future members of our club. I feel blessed to have had the opportunity to meet and become friends with literally thousands of people from our community and beyond, and I look forward to continuing this very special relationship I have with our members for years to come. Thank you for your continued support and the opportunity and pleasure to serve you over all of these years.

FOREWORD

I grew up in fitness. From not long after I was born up until this very day, I have been immersed in the fitness industry. At first I was involved as a spectator in the gym, since I was only a child tagging along with my parents, who owned and operated a health club. As I got older, I began reading on the subject of health and fitness, started working out in the gym, and went on to college, earning a diploma in Health and Fitness Promotions from Niagara College in Welland, Ontario as well as becoming a Certified Personal Trainer through the Canadian Society for Exercise Physiology. Today I have over fourteen years of experience in health and fitness, am currently certified by the American Council on Exercise as a personal trainer and have helped hundreds of people with their own health and fitness journeys.

Although I learned a lot from reading, and even more from my two-year college education, nothing comes close to what I gained from watching and listening to my father. His knowledge came from many years of real-world experience and real-world application working with real people. He has over thirty-five years of experience, so you'd better believe that there was a lot to learn and take away. I have seen him use his knowledge to help numerous people lose over one hundred pounds and several more lose fifty-plus pounds, to help people build muscle and compete in bodybuilding, and even to help someone get out of their wheelchair and walk on their own again. Amazing.

Lucky for you, my father wrote this book. As I did, you will learn from him everything you need to know to get started working out properly in the gym, right from what to bring up to what exercises to do, how to do them, and why. After reading this book you will no doubt be able to join a gym with confidence, knowing that you will get the most out of your workouts and maximize your results. Whether you are just starting out, have worked out before but had disappointing results, or are an experienced weightlifter, there is much to gain from reading this book.

The information in this book can change lives. A healthy lifestyle provides a higher quality of life. When you are strong and fit, you have more energy, more strength, and more confidence to take on anything you want. So, read this book, apply the information to your workouts, and enjoy life to its fullest.

Matthew Spada

ACKNOWLEDGEMENTS

Although I'm officially retired from the hustle and bustle of the rat race, I still, after thirty-five years, visit my health club frequently, mingle with the members, and check on everything, and I still look for opportunities to grow and/or improve the business. As I think back more and more about what I've accomplished and what all of those experiences have done for me, I can come to only one conclusion: my first acknowledgement should go to all of the past and present members of what is now my family's club. Without them, we'd have no business. They have stood by us through thick and thin.

Many of our members have been with us for over thirty years. The first member we ever signed up, on our first day of business back in May 1986, is still a member. To me, that speaks to the quality of the service we offer our community, and even more importantly, to the appreciation and continued support we have had from our dedicated members over all of these years. Because of this continued support, we have been able to sponsor many orphaned children from all corners of the globe and become monthly donors to Operation Smile and Sick Kids Hospital in Toronto, Ontario—all on behalf of and because of our members.

My second acknowledgement goes to my two wonderful children, Matthew and Stephanie, for their help with this book. Without it, this book would have been much more of a challenge than it was. Both are busy with their own lives: Matt, married with a wife and two children, has run my health club full-time for several years now, and Stephanie runs three of our dance retail stores and our online store single-handedly. They are both well-respected, mature, intelligent, responsible, hard-working adults, always there to help me out no matter how busy they are—just as I will always be there for them. It's the kind of relationship every parent hopes and prays for. I'm truly blessed. Thank you, Matt and Steph.

Gino A. Spada
Owner, G&M Fitness Ltd.
Since 1986

INTRODUCTION

One might ask how my obsession with strength training and fitness got started so many years ago. I'll just say that, for various reasons, it is important to some people to ensure that they never fall victim to ridicule, bullying, and abuse, especially in their youth. I took things into my own hands and made sure it didn't happen. I got in shape, stayed in shape, and didn't take any crap from anybody. That's me in a nutshell. It didn't take much because I have that nature about me that I enjoy working hard—physically hard—and challenging myself at every opportunity, whether it be sport or work. To this day, I rarely look for the easiest way to do things, physically speaking, so the allure of working out with weights and keeping fit and strong was interesting to me and rather appealing, right from a young age.

Being always alongside my mom and dad as a youngster when they were working around the house helped as well. They were immigrants from Italy and did everything themselves, manually—growing all of our food from an enormous garden; canning every fruit and vegetable known to humanity; curing; making sausage, spaghetti sauce, soppressata, capocollo, prosciutto, and olives; canning peaches, pears, peppers, and onions; making wine—you name it, I was there for it all. My dad even did his own concrete steps and sidewalks with his father at our home, and I was right there for that also.

I've come to the conclusion that all Italians are born with a few natural talents, a couple of which are the abilities to play soccer and mix cement.

Fast forward fifty years or so. I'm still in very good physical condition for my age, better than most; I still look forward to the physical challenge of any job I need to do; and I still don't take any crap from anyone—I'm always respectful, but never timid. If confrontation is what it takes for me to address an issue, then confrontation is what you're going to get—at least from me, anyway—face to face, no hiding behind a computer or text.

So, having said all that, I can imagine that you as the reader are beginning to understand already what kind of a book this is going to be. It's straight shooting, no bull; I say what I mean, and I mean what I say.

And now that you know me personally a bit better, let's get started.

I'd like to make a suggestion that helps me tremendously when I'm reading a book that I expect to learn something from—and you will definitely learn a few things from this book; I promise. So, get yourself a yellow highlighter. When you come across those "Aha!" moments, or those "Hey, that makes a lot of sense!" moments, or those "I didn't know that!" moments, or even those "I can't believe I've been doing that wrong all of these years!" moments, highlight them. Once you are done the book, you can go back and reread only the highlighted parts. By doing so, you'll ensure those newly learned concepts will have a better chance of not being forgotten. Also, doing the highlighting thing will allow you to go back to the book in the future and use the book as a quick reference and summary of all of the important things that you have learned from it. So, that's my only suggestion right now. I've also deliberately provided a blank "Notes" page at the end of each chapter for your convenience.

I wrote this book for two reasons. The first reason was to help people feel more confident and comfortable about deciding to finally join a health club. I realize health clubs can be very intimidating, and I also realize that this one obstacle—intimidation—keeps many people away from health clubs. That's very unfortunate. So, I came to the conclusion that if I provided enough information about what to expect, this information would somehow mitigate some of the anxiety and fear about simply walking into a health club and considering a membership.

The second reason I wrote this book was to try to better educate people about how to actually do the exercises properly. It never ceases to amaze me that even after thirty-five years operating my club and having trained literally thousands of people, I still, to this day, cannot walk through my club (or any other club, for that matter) without seeing members doing things incorrectly. I've scoured the aisles of many bookstores and have found nothing there that will do for you what this book will do.

I've worked out at clubs in Fort Myers, Florida; Varadero, Cuba; Rende, Italy; Montreal, Quebec; Baltimore, Maryland; Venice Beach, California; Toronto, Ontario; Stratford, Ontario; Hamilton, Ontario; Sarnia, Ontario; Cobourg, Ontario; Rochester, NY; Buffalo, NY; and others—so, I've been around. What aggravates me is that most of the time, it's the younger people making the mistakes—the ones who think that if they read a few articles, Google a few things, and talk to a few people with bigger muscles than them, they'll be all set to go. What's worse is that these young athletes will bring in one or both of their parents, who would be in their forties, fifties, or even their sixties, and show them everything they know without consulting a trainer. I've seen it first-hand in our club; the poor dad who listened to his son, rather than seek the advice of a good trainer, was pretty much bedridden for three or four days, very sore, swollen, and in a lot of pain. I just shake my head when I run across such occurrences.

If I had to stop and correct someone every time I saw someone doing something wrong as I walk through my own club, I would never get anywhere or get anything done. Now, don't get me wrong. At our club, we try very hard to offer what services we are able to provide, at every opportunity, free of charge, in an attempt to better educate our members. We offer free orientation to every member that first joins so that we can ensure that they get started on the right path, but if one thinks that they already know what they need to know, or knows someone who has been at it for a while, they'll elect to just go it on their own, or count on their friend or family member for guidance. Big mistake. For the most part, the older generation will seek help, but the younger generation won't. Today, everyone thinks all of the answers are online. In my opinion, too many are relying on Mr. Google for answers to questions that they should be seeking from an experienced professional, like me or my son!

Also, in an attempt to correct these mistakes, my son Matt and I offer several ongoing educational seminars at our club, which are also free and open to all members, but it's not working. Unfortunately, the ones making the mistakes don't realize they are making mistakes, so they don't attend the seminars.

So, this book is another attempt to better educate or inform those who have taken up weight training/strength training or wish to do so, and to provide the knowledge they require to help them join a health club with confidence and get the most out of their workouts. It is written for the beginners, the ones just starting out, although I personally know of many, many people who have been working out for years and still aren't doing things properly. So, this book is for anyone who intends to join a gym for the first time or who has already been a member of a gym for some time. They all will benefit in one way or another from the information in this book.

This book will take the reader on a step-by-step journey from how and where you should start, right through to being a confident, well-informed, knowledgeable member of any health club, anywhere. If one follows the advice in this book, I can assure you that he or she will be not the one asking questions of other members, but the one answering them.

Every word of advice I give in the following pages comes from over thirty-five years of experience and continuing education in the fitness field. In addition to my experience and credentials listed under "About the Author," I've read thousands of pages of research, old and new. But I find that all research is questioned or contradicted sooner or later, so in my mind, real-life experience trumps research every time. And real-life experience is what I have plenty of. Just because someone owns a health club for many years doesn't necessarily mean that they have experience, but in my small town, I not only owned the club, but I ran all of the day-to-day operations. I did the sign-ups, the consultations, the programming, the training, the hiring, the firing, the cleaning, the repairs—everything, every day, for years.

I have a lot to say in the following pages, so pay close attention, and don't discount what you are about to learn. You will learn some important things, regardless of what stage you are at in your training; trust me.

Sit back, relax, take your time through this book, reread as is necessary, and enjoy it, as it has a lot to offer. I can promise you this one thing: by the time you have read this entire book and absorbed what it has to say, you will at the very least be able to do one thing for certain, and that's to **START RIGHT!**

CHAPTER 1:
Why Join a Gym?

Good question! I guess I'd better make this a good answer, because let's face it: isn't that what this book is all about? Truth be told, I sat for hours attempting to express in words why I feel so strongly about getting as many individuals as possible to join a health club. Well, here it is.

IMPROVED QUALITY OF LIFE

One reason you should join a health club (as soon as you finish reading this book, of course) is that once you introduce regular strength training and cardiovascular training into your life as this book describes, you will inevitably improve not only your physical self but your mental self, and in doing so, will achieve a much higher quality of life than you would expect. Let me explain what I mean by that last part.

Most people in modern society simply accept the fact that as they get older, their physical abilities will diminish. Well, I'm here to tell you that although some physical decline is expected, too many expect it much sooner in their lives than they should. It's because they don't realize how they should feel at, say, sixty or seventy or even eighty years old. They don't realize how much strength they are losing prematurely by not using and challenging their muscles often enough as they age. The old adage, "Use it or lose it," cannot be more accurate.

I'll use myself as an example. Keep in mind that I am sixty years old as I write this. Do I feel that I am unable to physically do what I could do when I was in high school because of my age? No. Do I feel that I am not as strong as I was when I was in my twenties and thirties? No. Do I feel that I am less mentally sharp now than I was in my twenties and thirties? No. I honestly don't feel any different now at sixty than when I was much younger. Not much has changed. Why? Because I joined a health club when I was nineteen, and I have been strength training regularly since I was sixteen; that's why. I'm sure that those reading this that are my age, or a bit younger or even a bit older, are thinking, "Well, it's probably too late for me now," and that's not the case at all. As a matter of fact, the changes you will realize by introducing regular strength training into your life at a senior age will amaze you. It's because you have a lot more to gain—or regain, in your case, at a more senior age—than someone who is very young. The young crowd has not had to deal with the consequences of aging, but you have, and much of that can be reversed if not eliminated altogether. If you are my age and "feel old," you are doing yourself an enormous disservice by not joining a health club. So, read this book, and then go join that club and change your life forever.

LIFE GETS EASIER

Another good reason, and the one that can be realized only if you incorporate the suggestions in this book into your life consistently, is that once you make it a priority to take care of yourself in one way or another each day, the day and what seem like its never-ending challenges become easier to handle.

HEALTH CLUB OR HOME?

Not to sound self-serving, but in my experience, I cannot say that I've come across anyone who can honestly say they are more content with their workouts and results at home than if they were at a gym. Unless you are like me and would rather be alone when you work out, have a lot of self-motivation, knowledge, and experience, and have more equipment at home than you can shake a stick at (like me), you'll never be able to accomplish with your home gym what you can in a well-equipped, well-run health club (like mine!).

NOTES

CHAPTER 2:
When Can I Start?

Before you run out and join a gym, there is one thing (besides reading this book)—and the only thing, in my mind—that should keep you from doing just that: your age. The next statement you are going to read is by far the most valid one you are going to read in this book, and here it is:

You can certainly be too young to join a gym and take up serious strength training, but you can *never* be too old.

This question of when you should start is directly related to the stage of physical development you are at. If you are over the age of sixteen, it's irrelevant. Get started. If you are younger than sixteen, the stage of your physical development is the determining factor. I've seen some fifteen-year-olds that look physically like they are twelve, and I've seen other fifteen-year-olds that look like they are eighteen. Everyone is different, everyone develops at different speeds, and that's why I'm such a fan of personal training. Personal trainers treat every client as an individual with their own unique set of circumstances, issues, challenges, abilities, and so on. So, if you are reading this book and you are younger than sixteen, I would strongly suggest you start with body weight exercises only, such as push-ups, sit-ups, and chin-ups. That's all you need. Do them every day. Once you reach the age of sixteen, you should be ready to start a basic strength training program with weight resistance. If you are a parent eager to get your child stronger for a particular sport, please heed my advice and don't jump the gun. A thirteen-year-old child should not be lifting weights.

I've experienced many times the persistence of a parent or parents to get their young child into weight training too early to "toughen them up" or "get them stronger" in an attempt to help them excel in their sport. These parents show up at the gym, their thirteen-year-old child beside them, insisting that they should be lifting weights. But there are still natural growth mechanisms in play in that young body that should not be interrupted by premature, unnecessary, repetitive overload on the bones, muscles, tendons, and ligaments.

HOW YOUNGSTERS SHOULD START

Here's how I started and how I would like you to consider starting if you are fifteen or younger. Although I was very active and athletic in school, I really didn't start working out with weights until I was about seventeen, and I didn't join a health club until I was nineteen. I started with chin-ups (or pull-ups, as they are referred to by some), push-ups, and sit-ups. That's what I recommend to those parents who want to get their kids into weight training too early. Body weight exercises are all they need at this point. I did those exercises consistently, day after day. At the age of seventeen, I could perform several hundred sit-ups without any problem, I did seventy-five push-ups without missing a beat and actually had to have someone place weight plates on my back after a while to create more resistance, and did twenty to thirty chins with no problem—along with skipping (I can skip like a boxer to this day), jogging, biking, ball hockey, ice hockey, soccer, volleyball, basketball, gymnastics, and track and field, all at school. That stuff alone got me into very good physical condition without lifting any weights at all. Eventually I purchased a bench press for the basement and a set of barbells and dumbbells. I stuck with basic bench pressing for my upper body, one-arm rows for my back, bar curls, and tricep extensions, and continued with the other stuff at school. In grades eleven and twelve, I started using the school's weight room at lunch breaks consistently and got into even better shape lifting weights—although, thinking back, I realize I made all of the classic mistakes that all young people make when starting out. If I had had a book like this to read prior to beginning training in my school gym, I would have been much further ahead leaving high school. I graduated from high school and went to work in a factory at eighteen years of age. I joined my first gym with a friend at the age of nineteen.

So, don't be in a hurry to join a gym if you are still developing and growing on your own. In my opinion, do what I did until you are at least sixteen; then, as long as you've read and understood the information in this book, you have my blessing. Join with confidence.

HOW NEWBIES SHOULD START

If you haven't done any weight training before, regardless of your age, you're reading the right book. Most people I see, especially younger people, learn what to do and how to do it from watching others, asking others, reading magazines, and so on. Well, if you want to do something the right way, learn from someone who has already done it and been successful. That's me!

If you are at the right age or even at that ripe old age, get to it. As I mentioned earlier, you can never be too old to join a gym and take up regular exercise, and more specifically effective strength training. I know what a lot of you in your senior years and even younger are thinking: "I've never worked out in a gym, let alone do any kind of physical exercise in my life," or, "I have ailments that are keeping me from exercising."

DON'T LET HEALTH CONDITIONS HOLD YOU BACK

Here's some of what I've heard over the years from people who are just looking for an excuse not to join a gym and take up exercise—or, in most cases, who simply lack knowledge or awareness of how beneficial regular exercise can be for them regardless of their physical condition or know-how. I've heard: I can't work out because I have arthritis, I have high blood pressure, I have fibromyalgia, I have diabetes, I have a bad back, I have depression, I have cancer, I'm legally blind, I'm in a wheelchair, and so on.

Well, I'm here to tell you that although these are all valid concerns, any good doctor will tell you that the more physically fit you are, the better chance you have to not only better cope with or manage these kinds of conditions, but some you may be able to overcome altogether. More and more doctors are seeing the research that proves beyond a shadow of a doubt that eating well and taking up regular exercise are the keys to well-being and improved health, not to mention that it certainly makes their job a lot easier. The valid research is out there, so if you don't believe me, look it up for yourself.

The reason I mentioned those specific conditions above is that I've dealt with every one of them over the years as the primary trainer in my gym and have seen the almost miraculous results that good, effective, regular exercise can provide—and, more specifically, effective strength training. It will change your life.

Just for fun, here are some of the excuses that I don't accept and usually just ignore, along with a few thoughts that go through my head when I hear them:

"I don't have time." (My thought: "We are open 24/7. How much more time do you need?")

"I'm embarrassed." (My thought: "Get over yourself. No one is here to look at you.")

"I have to get in shape first before I join." (My thought: "What?")

"I can't afford it." (My thought—and I say this one out loud: "We can make it work for you. We turn away no one. What can you afford?")

"I'm too tired after work." (My thought: "You are too tired after work because you are not exercising.")

Like I said at the beginning of this book, you'll get no bull from me.

So, carry on and continue with the next chapters, which will outline not only all stages of weight resistance training, from beginner's basic exercises to the most advanced, but, just as importantly, the kinds of things that you should be aware of prior to even stepping inside a gym for the first time. You'll find that as you continue to read, your confidence level will rise, you'll begin to feel as if you will not be so lost and unprepared in a new gym setting, and you will develop a new eagerness to take that first step and walk into that gym.

My hope is that this will be the case; if it is after reading this book, I feel that I've done my job. Read on, take notes, and prepare yourself for what will be one of the most important things you will ever do in your lifetime, and that's to join a gym.

NOTES

CHAPTER 3:
What to Expect When You Join a Gym

So, it's time. Whether you were underage, have done what I outlined for you to do in chapter 2, and are now of age; you are in fairly good physical condition; you are a bit more knowledgeable; or it's just the right time for you in your life to finally join a gym—congratulations! You're about to conquer the hardest step—simply showing up at the gym for the first time. I'm going to walk you through this one step by step.

It'll be a bit intimidating at first because likely you'll be the only one standing there with hands in pocket while everyone else is working out, but keep a stiff upper lip; it's no big deal; hang in there. Realize that everyone on that gym floor has done exactly what you are doing at one time or another.

Hopefully, wherever you are, there is a really nice gym (like mine) that has friendly, knowledgeable, and accommodating staff awaiting your arrival.

WALKING INTO A GYM FOR THE FIRST TIME

Upon arrival, utter these words and these words only, to the front desk staff: "Hello, I'd like to try your gym." That's all you should have to say. If the front desk staff start talking about considering a paid membership right away, their job is likely to pass you on to a salesperson who will sit you in an office and attempt to sign you up for a membership right then and there. Decline to listen; here's why.

What should happen, and it happens at our club, is that they should offer you a free, or close to free, trial period (like my gym does) with no commitment to join, simply because you are a first-time visitor. Make sure in the preliminary paperwork that you will be asked to sign that there is no commitment to join afterwards, and do not give them any payment information. At this point in time, there is no reason for that. This paperwork should be some sort of liability waiver protecting the gym against a lawsuit if you get hurt and an opportunity for you to inform the gym of any and all health issues or concerns that you may have at the time.

Some gyms will automatically place you into a paying membership after your trial period is over unless you cancel, so beware of that. Read the entire copy before you sign, and if there is anything in there that I've warned you about, have them cross out what you don't want in there, or just refuse to sign it. Just be ready to be refused and sent home. Hopefully, if that happens, there is another gym around that you can check out.

If they've done the right thing and offered you a chance to try out the gym with a free or sweet introductory offer like we have in place, once you've done the paperwork, you're in. Next, you should ask the staff if there is any kind of an orientation included with your trial. Hopefully (again), there is (like there is at my club!).

If not, no worries—you've read the book, and although it will take some getting used to the strange environment, you'll be fine; trust me. Depending on how they monitor attendance, you may be given a membership card, a swipe card, an ID badge, or something similar. Don't lose it. Also, don't let them upsell you on using additional amenities like the swimming pool, classes, or personal training. You are there to check out their gym, do some basic strength training, and nothing else right now. "No, thank you," would be the correct response to any of those types of offers when you first join.

Hopefully (yet again), the accommodating staff will show you around the facility so you can become a bit more comfortable with the locations of the kinds of things you are looking for. Don't be afraid to ask if you don't see a certain machine or apparatus you would like to use in your workout. Perhaps a good idea would be to bring a list of machines you would want to use and look for them on your walk-though.

Make sure that when you do decide to actually go to the gym to look for this type of trial you are not in a hurry. This would be the time to ask questions of the staff and look around for things like the bulletin board, the rules, and member notices. Not all gyms are run the same way, and all have different rules regarding things like what you can and can't wear, gym etiquette, shoes, gym bags, cardio time limits, and sanitary rules, so take your time and have a really good look around before you leave or before you change for your first workout.

There you have it. You've done it. You are now a member of a health club. Congrats again because this will likely be one of the smartest decisions you've ever made for yourself.

NOTES

CHAPTER 4:
What to Wear and What to Bring

Let's assume that this is a new experience for you. The following is a complete list of what you should consider bringing with you to the gym. Some things are mandatory, and some are optional, depending on your particular situation. I'll try to cover them all.

THE GYM BAG

First and foremost, get yourself a gym bag. The club you have joined may even have their own branded gym bags for sale (like we do at our club), so consider that first. I say that because now that you are a member of this club, you have to keep in mind that in one way or another, you should always consider supporting that club, whether it is by purchasing a drink once in a while, or buying a T-shirt or gym bag. What irritates me to no end is the member who joins our club only when there is some sort of discount (which, by the way, we don't do anymore), brings their own drink and protein bar from home that they bought at Costco, carries a gym bag from Walmart, and wears a T-shirt from some other gym. What's even worse is that some ask us for permission to use our cooler to keep their post-workout drink cold while they work out. The post-workout drink they bought somewhere else! Nice. Thanks for the support! The other thing to keep in mind is that in most cases (ours being one of them), the gym will likely be the cheapest place to purchase any branded products because they are not interested in making a bunch of profit from these items; rather, they like to see people wearing or carrying a product around town with their logo on them.

The gym bag is important because you need to have a good, supportive, clean, and dry pair of runners just for the gym, especially if you live in a climate that is not always clean and dry. The worst thing you can do is show up at the gym in your runners after you've worn them outside through the snow, rain, slush, and what have you, and head right for the change rooms and gym floor without changing into a clean, dry pair of shoes. Take it from me: the staff will take offence, and I don't blame them for one second. That's inconsiderate and uncalled for.

Second, another reason you should have a gym bag is that if you sweat (and you should), you should have a place to put your sweaty clothes after your workout and shower, and a place to put your wet towel and clean gym shoes. If you choose to shower at home, great (saves me money), but you still need that gym bag for other things: hygiene products, personal belongings like your phone, wallet, cash, and jewelry, your membership card or swipe card, and a lock of some kind so you can lock it up in a locker while you are working out.

COMFORTABLE THREADS

Comfortable workout clothing is essential. You must be comfortable, fresh, and clean. Use garments that are either one hundred percent cotton or some sort of high-tech material made exclusively for workouts that supposedly wicks away sweat and helps keep you cooler. All gyms are different as to temperature inside the facility. I've worked out in gyms that are way too cold and also in gyms that are way too hot. You'll have to play it by ear for a few workouts to be able to determine how much or how little clothing to be wearing during your workout. And, speaking of how little—don't be a hero and wear a muscle shirt that barely covers your upper body. Trust me; it looks ridiculous, and most decent clubs don't allow them anyway. Cut-off sleeves, sure, but better yet, stick with just a clean T-shirt; you'll be safer that way. And pick a T-shirt that doesn't have derogatory statements or profanity on it. That's not appreciated. The last thing you want to do is bring attention to yourself because of something you've done or something you've worn that has irritated or upset another member. Got it? Good.

Forget the cologne or perfume. In most public gathering places these days, use of fragrance is frowned upon anyway.

That list should get you started.

NOTES

CHAPTER 5:
Gym Etiquette

I think that once you've read through this chapter, you should feel more at ease in the gym because you'll have a better understanding of what is expected of you as a member of that particular club and how you are expected to conduct yourself while you are there. Remember: all clubs are run differently, so don't assume that the rules in one club are the same in all others. Some of this stuff is just common sense, and some needs a bit of explaining. Oddly enough, they are all issues that we have had to address in our club at one time or another, so here we go.

FRESH THREADS

As I mentioned in chapter 4, always wear clean, fresh workout clothes. You don't want to be the one wearing the same shorts and T-shirt every workout, especially if they are wrinkled. That just screams, "I just pulled these clothes out of my gym bag from the last workout." If you wear workout gloves, be forewarned that the constant sweat from your hands will sooner or later cause those gloves to stink like crazy because nobody ever thinks to wash them. If you use them, wash them periodically, please.

OCCUPIED EQUIPMENT

In regard to using the equipment in the gym, there will inevitably be two situations that you will come across that you need to know how to handle. The first is when you want to use a machine that is being used by another member doing multiple sets, sitting on the machine between sets, talking too much, or whatever. In most cases, people hate to wait around to use a machine that is already being used. It interrupts their workout and makes their time in the gym a lot longer, or they choose to not wait and skip it altogether.

Here's what to do if you want to use that occupied machine. Go over to the member using the machine and ask politely if you can "work in." That's it. If the member you are asking knows anything about gym etiquette, he or she will let you work in. By working in, you will alternate sets. You do a set, they do a set, and so on. If they say no, or ask you to wait, just walk away. Now, having said that, if you are the one using the machine and another member asks you if they can "work in," the answer should always be, "Sure." You do a set, they do a set, you do a set, and they do a set. Everyone's happy. That's how it should work, so don't be a jerk.

WHAT COMES OUT OF YOUR MOUTH

No profanity. The gym is a public place like all others, and there's no place for profanity. If you are one of those who use profanity in casual conversation with your friends, be careful to avoid it at the gym because you are almost always in earshot of another member who will overhear you. Think about that. You may think it makes you seem tough or macho or cool in some way, but it doesn't. If you don't have anything nice to say, just keep your mouth shut, and do your workout.

EQUIPMENT USE

Don't drop the weights on the floor or slam the weight stack at the end of your set (for an explanation of the term "weight stack," see chapter 7). Control every inch of every movement. Dropping weights is the same as using profanity. The only attention you'll get is the kind you don't want, and I'll be addressing the importance of control in chapter 9.

In most gyms (like ours), if you have used a machine and are sweating on it, you are expected to spray and wipe down that machine when you are done with it. There should be several cleaning stations throughout the gym that supply paper towels and disinfectant cleaner to do just that. If there isn't, there should be! Cleaning up properly after you sweat on a machine is common courtesy. No one wants to deal with someone else's sweat.

KEEPING THE GOOD VIBE

This last one is not etiquette, but if you do it, it will be much appreciated by the staff; most people don't do this one. This little thing makes an owner/operator or a full-time front desk staff member feel really good. It has happened to me several times, and it just makes me feel appreciated for all the hard work in running the business. It's a simple little thing but makes a huge impression, especially if you mean it. It's two simple words: "Thank you." Rather than saying "Good-bye" or "Have a nice day" as you are walking out of the club past the front desk on your way out, say "Thank you" instead. Trust me when I tell you it makes a tremendous impression on the staff. Now, I'm assuming that your club is a good one (like mine) and there is actually something to be thankful for. If you are not happy with the way the club is run and the staff is unpleasant and inattentive, and the place is a dump, then "Good-bye" may be more appropriate.

NOTES

CHAPTER 6:
Monkey See, Monkey Do

I have to admit, once I concocted a made-up exercise, just for fun, something no one had ever seen before, and performed it in the gym for a few weeks to prove a point. You can imagine what happened. After a few weeks there were numerous members (monkeys) doing the same exercise. They had no idea what it did, how effective it was, or why they should do it. They just saw me doing it and assumed they should too. I guess maybe I should take that as a compliment. They assumed I knew what I was doing, so it must be good. The point is, if you really don't know why someone is doing something unfamiliar or performing an exercise differently than how you've been taught (assuming you've been taught properly), don't assume you should do it or change what you're doing because chances are, you'll be heading down the wrong road.

DON'T WATCH

I tell everyone when they start, "Don't watch other people!" There are many different reasons why someone might be doing an exercise differently than how you've been taught—perhaps lack of flexibility, injuries, or lack of knowledge. Learn the correct way to perform the exercises that you will be doing (we're going to do that for you, so don't worry), and just do them as you've been taught. We also have a series of videos for you to watch (see chapter 10) that demonstrate exactly how to do the exercises properly. Talk about spoon-feeding, eh? Like I said in the beginning, this book and the information you'll get from it are all you are going to need. You're going to be so smart!

On the other hand, while working out at other gyms, I've seen members performing exercises that I'd never seen before and found to be quite impressive, so upon my return to my own gym, I started doing those myself, and lo and behold, after a few weeks, they became commonplace. But in those cases, I brought to light a certain exercise that was beneficial and could easily be incorporated into anyone's workout, and for good reason.

I can watch an exercise being performed and be able to figure out whether it would be effective. In your case, you likely don't have the knowledge or expertise yet to figure that out for yourself, so just don't do it. Furthermore, you don't know where these members discovered these exercises and whether they even know what they are doing.

And remember this one if you are a young man or woman just starting out: "Big muscles don't necessarily mean big brains." Don't assume if you see a member with big muscles that what they say is bible, because in a lot of cases, it's not—and you know as well as I do that there are several ways to build big muscles besides working out properly, if you know what I mean.

NOTES

CHAPTER 7:
Know the Terminology

Reps, sets, positive contractions, negative contractions, muscle failure, drop sets, spotting, split routines, anatomically correct positioning, wrist wraps versus wrist straps, flexion and extension, selectorized machines, weight stacks—the list goes on and on. We'll cover the ones that I feel are commonplace, the ones I feel you'll come across more often than not in conversation with a trainer or other members.

REPS

The two terms "reps" and "sets" are the ones that most beginners get confused or reversed. "Reps" (or "repetitions") refers to the number of times you lift the weight up and down, out and in, whatever the case may be, without stopping until you can't do another lift or "repetition" with good form.

SETS

The "set" refers to the group of repetitions you perform at one time. So, if you are performing a bench press, you pick up the bar with the correct grip position, lower it to your chest, press it up, and repeat until you have to return it or "rack" it. That is considered one "set." So, if you pressed that weight ten times before stopping, you've done one "set" of ten "repetitions" or "reps."

POSITIVE AND NEGATIVE CONTRACTIONS

"Positive" and "negative" contractions describe the muscles' movement while lifting. The best and simplest example I can give that illustrates this perfectly is the standing bicep curl. If you are standing, holding a barbell in your hands, when you lift or "curl" the barbell up to your chest, the bicep muscles must "shorten" or "contract" in order to bend or "flex" the elbow to lift the weight up. That is the first phase of the lift, and it is referred to as the "positive contraction." When you let the bar back down with control to the starting position, those same bicep muscles needs to "lengthen" again in order to allow the elbow to "extend" back to the straight-arm position. It's almost like they are working as a brake to give you control as you bring the load back to the start position. That is the "negative contraction." In summary, the "positive contraction" is when the working muscle shortens, and the "negative contraction" is when the working muscle lengthens.

MUSCLE FAILURE

"Muscle failure" is when you get to the maximum number of repetitions that you can do without losing your form. You have then completed a set of repetitions to "muscle failure," which means you cannot do another repetition with proper form. Good job!

FLEXION AND EXTENSION

We have already touched on "flexion" and "extension" in the standing barbell curl example above. When you lift the bar, the bicep muscles contract or shorten to bend the elbow joint; this is "flexion" of the elbow joint. When you lower the bar back down, the bicep muscle lengthens so "extension" of the elbow is possible. In other words, bending or collapsing a joint by way of a positive contraction of a working muscle or muscles is referred to as "flexion," while straightening a joint by way of a negative contraction of a working muscle or muscles is referred to as "extension."

You can also do a positive contraction of a muscle to extend a joint. For example, in the tricep extension (for a description of this exercise, see Chapter 10), you are doing a positive contraction or shortening the tricep muscles against a load to extend the elbow joint.

SPLIT ROUTINE

Usually, when we start a beginner out in strength training, we start with a full-body routine. We incorporate all of the basic exercises that address all of the major muscle groups in the body. Because proper rest and recuperation between workouts is necessary for optimal results, we highly recommend that the full-body workout not be done on consecutive days, because once you work a certain muscle group, you need enough rest to ensure that you have fully recovered prior to working it again. Here's where the term "split routine" comes in. Once you've done the full-body workout for a few months, you are going to want to strength train more often than just two or three days a week, and you will likely be ready to add more exercises per body part. The solution is to break up your routine so that you have two or more different workouts, each addressing one or more (but not all) muscle groups; you can now work out on consecutive days and do more exercises per body part, working only two or three body parts per workout. Those routines are referred to as "split routines" because you've essentially taken your full-body workout and split it up into two or more workouts. It may be upper body one day and lower body the next. It may be all pushing movements one day and pulling movements the next. More on that in Bonus Chapter 3.

SPOTTING

First off, if someone asks you to "spot" them and you don't know how to do it properly, don't! The spotter is the person who stands by while the lifter does his or her set, and the lifter expects a bit of help with the last few repetitions at the end of the set. This takes know-how and experience. I've seen this go very wrong many times in our own gym. More on that in chapter 8.

SELECTORIZED MACHINES

"Selectorized" means the level of resistance is adjusted by moving a pin or lever.

WEIGHT STACK

The "weight stack" refers to the stack of weight plates that are already attached to a machine where the user can simply place a selector pin in the desired weight plate, rather than having to load free weight plates on the machine and then remove them when you are done.

DROP SETS

This type of training is not seen a lot anymore, but is still a valid and effective way of training, although it can be done only sporadically because it takes so much out of the person and the muscle being trained. A drop set is done by performing several sets of the same exercise without any rest between sets, and the sets get lighter and lighter as you go. The purpose of this type of training is to fatigue as many muscle fibres as possible. Allow me to explain. When you do a normal set to muscle failure, all that means is that the muscle or muscles involved cannot do another repetition properly because you have fatigued enough fibres to bring that muscle to failure, so you are done. There are not enough fresh muscle fibres left to lift that same weight again. But, if you were to do another set with a lighter weight, you would still be able to lift for more repetitions using the remaining muscle fibres that have not been brought to failure. To illustrate, let's take the bicep curl as an example again. We would typically line up several pre-loaded bars on the floor. The first one would be the heaviest—let's say an eighty-pound bar. Then, perhaps, a fifty-pound bar, then a thirty-pound bar, and lastly a twenty-pound bar. You would stand between the first and second bar, pick up the first bar, perform as many reps as you could properly, and set it down. You would then, without resting, proceed to the next (lighter) bar, and then to the next, and then to the next. By the time you got to the last (lightest) bar, you would barely be able to do even a few repetitions because you had fatigued pretty much all of the muscle fibres in the muscle or muscles necessary to perform that lift. The same can be done on a selectorized machine. The spotter pulls the pin out of the weight stack when you are done your first heavy set and places it at a lighter setting for the next set, and so on until you are not able to do any more reps, even with a very light weight. Cool, eh?

ANATOMICALLY CORRECT POSITIONING

"Anatomically correct positioning" describes the proper position for your body to be in, in order to allow natural movement and isolation of the muscles you are working in order to reap the most benefit from the exercise.

WRIST WRAPS AND WRIST STRAPS

These tend to get confused a lot. The "wrist wrap" is added support for your wrist. It wraps around the wrist. The "wrist strap" is to help with your grip. It goes around your wrist when you are lifting very heavy weights and then goes around the bar or dumbbell that you are lifting in order to help you hang on longer.

There's more, but if you're a beginner, becoming familiar with the ones I've listed above will get you off to a great start.

NOTES

CHAPTER 8:
Tips For a Great Workout

This is the ultimate "dos and don'ts" list that will inevitably result in a more efficient and effective workout. Some tips may sound trivial, but they are important. I've based most of this chapter on a seminar I offer at my club called "The 8 Biggest Mistakes in Strength Training, Body Building, and Power Lifting," and all of the advice comes from my training experience over the last thirty-five years.

FOCUS

There are so many distractions these days that it is almost impossible to focus or concentrate on the task at hand without interruption. If you are serious about results, leave your phone turned off or locked up in a locker with your gear. Don't bring a magazine with you into the workout area so you can read between sets—ridiculous. If you get motivated by a certain type of music, then by all means use an MP3 and ear buds. Ear buds will also keep most people from striking up a friendly yet interruptive conversation with you in the middle of your workout. When you are training, your focus should be on your muscles and how they feel, your form, and nothing else. More on focus in chapter 16.

PARTNERS

Having a partner can be a great thing. If they are a good partner, they should be able to keep you motivated and consistent. There's nothing better than having someone there beside you while you are performing your set, cheering you on with positive encouragement. Here's the thing, though—and this comes from personal experience: always prepare yourself for a great workout with or without your partner. Arrive at the gym with the mindset that you will begin a great workout at the scheduled time whether your partner is there or not. If you rely too much on a partner being there with you, the day will come when that partnership will end, or they just won't show up one day without letting you know, and you find yourself on your own. If you have the mindset I mentioned above, none of that will matter. Like I state in my seminar, "The best thing you can do is find yourself a partner, and the worst thing you can do is rely on a partner."

PROPER FORM

Be a stickler for proper form, just like me. That's one thing I was known for in my gym when I worked out there. Everyone, especially my partners, would comment on how strict I was with my form on each and every rep of each and every set. I accepted nothing less than perfect form, always. I have a saying when I'm training someone in regard to form, and it goes like this: "Your last heaviest rep of your last heaviest set should look no different than your first lightest rep of your first lightest set." Nothing should change. If your body position changes near the end as you struggle to do a few last reps, you are wasting your time and effort and increasing your risk of injury. Don't do those reps.

OVERTRAINING

The human body is a wonderful thing. It will adapt to pretty much anything we throw at it in an effort to survive and thrive. Adaptation occurs while resting. If you don't give your body enough time to fully recuperate from a tough workout, classic overtraining will occur, and your results will suffer—not to mention you will likely suffer an injury and not realize why. In weightlifting or bodybuilding, more is not necessarily better. I trained legs once a week for years with outstanding results. Once a week, one exercise: squats. Again from personal experience: consistency is the key, not pounding yourself into submission day after day. More on that in chapters 12 and 15!

LIGHTER WEIGHT, MORE REPETITIONS

Here's something you are going to hear in the gym sooner or later—I guarantee it: "I'm going to trim down so I'm doing more reps and less weight." This is one of the biggest misconceptions in pretty much every gym: that if you lighten up on the weight, that in turn allows you to do more repetitions and thus burn more calories, resulting in weight loss. Nothing can be further from the truth. Although you will burn more calories because of the extra repetitions per set, the effect on actual fat loss is negligible. Always, always, always lift to muscle failure, between six and twelve reps. Lifting lighter weights that you are already quite able to handle does not place any kind of necessary challenge or load on your muscles to result in muscle gain. You are doing strength training to get stronger, so there's only one way to do that, and that's to overload your muscles, not under load them. I would go so far as to say that this type of training, with lighter weights than you would normally train with, would be considered "active rest." Active rest definitely has a place. If, for instance, you've been training very hard for several months and just feel you need a bit of a break, but you don't want to stop altogether, then perhaps a week or two with lighter weights is just what the doctor ordered.

WARM UP

Always warm up before you start lifting. Hop on any cardio machine, and use it at a high enough intensity and/or speed to break a sweat. This should take no more than five minutes. There are many things that happen inside your body as a result of a good, effective warm-up. Many natural mechanisms are triggered to prepare the body for a physical challenge ahead. The heart starts pumping much faster, thus sending more oxygenated blood to your extremities faster. In the major joints like your hip joints and shoulder joints, there are small sacks of lubrication called synovial sacs that excrete—you guessed it—synovial fluid, to pre-lubricate those joints in preparation for the challenge ahead. Like I said, the human body is a wonderful thing, and these types of mechanisms are in place all over your body to help protect you against injury. So, don't be a slouch when warming up, and don't let anyone tell you it's not necessary. Just ask any professional athlete how important a good warm-up is.

CONTROL YOUR LIFTING

I've dedicated chapter 9 to this one, so stand by—it's that important.

NOTES

CHAPTER 9:
Proper Form

This is a big one and a very important one, so pay attention. This is the stuff I've been preaching to my clients for over thirty-five years. These instructions never change. They are the basic knowledge you need in order to be successful in your workouts and see the best results. They are the Golden Rules. Let's get started.

Would you jump into a deep lake without a life jacket before you learned how to swim, or would you learn how to swim first and then jump into the lake? It's the same with joining a gym. Do you think it would be beneficial to learn how to perform the exercises you are going to do prior to joining, especially if all of the information you need can be found in a book, just like the one you have in your hands right now? That's what chapter 10 is going to do for you. You are going to read about how to do these exercises, what the proper form should look like, and why—and you will also be provided with access to our video series that illustrates how to perform all of the necessary exercises you'll likely begin with to get you started in the right way. By the time you are done with chapter 10, you will not need to ask anyone how to use the equipment in your gym, or how to properly perform pretty much any exercise. You will recognize which exercises to do, whether on a machine or with free weights, whether they are basic movements or advanced, and so on. You'll be an expert before you start.

UNTIL YOU'RE SIXTEEN

As mentioned in chapter 2, if you are an adolescent, younger than sixteen, eager to be bigger, stronger, and faster than your friends, trust me when I tell you that all you need at this stage in your life are body weight exercises. In my opinion, push-ups are number one. If I had to pick one exercise that I thought would be the most effective, beneficial, full-body exercise without using weights, it would be the push-up. Add sit-ups and chin-ups (or pull-ups, as some call them, or sometimes "chins"), and you're all set. Do them regularly, every day if you can, and let your natural body functions develop you as they are meant to at that age, without disruption. Your skeletal structure is developing on its own at this point and should not be disrupted. Once you are about sixteen or so, we'll hit the weights, so those preliminary body weight exercises will better prepare you for that. So, be patient.

Once you are of age, sixteen or so, and you've prepared yourself physically by doing your push-ups, sit-ups, and chins as I recommended, you will be ready to hit the weights. You will stick to the basics and only the basics because they are the foundation of any exercise routine—regardless of how advanced you are or think you are. After over forty years of training, I still do the basics regularly. Some things are just too important to not do. So, here we go with the basics, one exercise at a time. In chapter 10, I'll tell you what it is, what it will do for you, and how to perform it with perfect form.

AFTER YOU'VE REACHED THE AGE OF SIXTEEN

If you are already of age or even much older and you've never weight trained before, same thing—start with the following basics.

FIRST THINGS FIRST—CONTROL

There are two things I would like to mention before getting into the exercises and the proper form. These are the things that you should keep in mind with absolutely every exercise that you do so I don't have to keep repeating them every time I describe an exercise, which I likely will do anyway because they are so important.

First, always, always, always be in control of the movement. No swinging, no thrusting, no twisting and struggling to gain an extra repetition—just slow, controlled movements lifting and lowering back to the start position. Got it? More on that coming up.

WORKING TO MUSCLE FAILURE

Secondly, you need to perform every set to what's called "muscle failure." What that means is that you should be working with enough resistance (weight) that allows you to perform only ten to twelve repetitions with proper form. If you tried to do more, you would have to cheat. Now, if you are new to weight training, obviously, you should not train to muscle failure right away. Give yourself a chance to get used to the exercise before challenging yourself with more resistance. Once you feel confident that you are doing the exercise correctly and need more of a challenge, then start to increase the weight until you find the weight that gets you to muscle failure somewhere between ten and twelve repetitions. Use common sense here when you are increasing the weight load. It is much safer to choose a weight that is too light than to choose a weight that is too heavy and risk injury. Got it? Great.

NOTES

CHAPTER 10:
Start with the Basics

Okay, now that we got those two important things, control and muscle failure, out of the way, let's keep them both in mind and move on to the actual basic exercises and how to do them properly.

Be prepared to spend a fair bit of time on this chapter. Each exercise description below contains introductory information to explain the purpose and orient you; a summary of the muscles and muscle groups involved; and a guide to correct technique and proper form.

ADJUSTING EQUIPMENT

As you approach any exercise machine, stand back and check to see what sections of the machine are adjustable. Most machines have adjustments for seat height, perhaps a chest pad to position your body relevant to the rest of the machine, etc. With the correct adjustments you should feel very comfortable performing the movement and feel that you are moving in a natural way.

USE THIS BOOK WITH OUR VIDEOS

In order to really grasp and learn from this "how to" chapter, for each exercise you should read the description and then immediately go to the video. I'm confident that with both the written description and the video, it will all make sense. So, here we go.

BENCH PRESS, DUMBBELL PRESS, AND VERTICAL CHEST PRESS

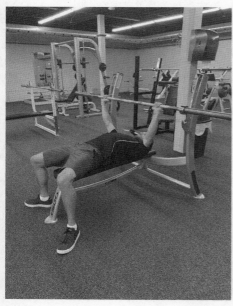
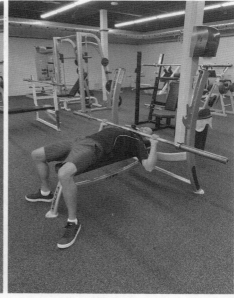

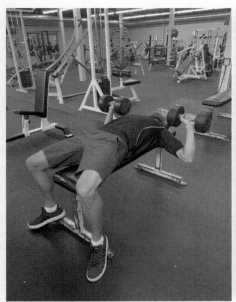 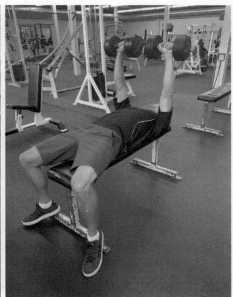

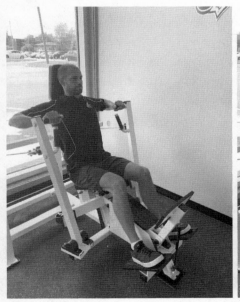 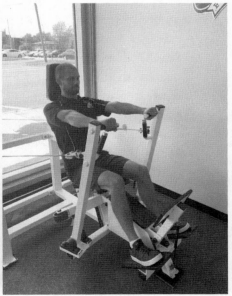

Introduction—Push-Ups Plus

I've grouped these three variations of the chest press together because they all do the same thing, and depending on your age, experience, and fitness level, you can pick the one you prefer. Most older adults or first-timers would choose the vertical chest press, as you are in a comfortable, seated position rather than lying back on a bench as with the other two, and the vertical chest press is done on a machine with a selectorized weight stack rather than using free weights, which the other two involve.

These three exercises mimic the push-up, with a difference: they allow you to gradually add more weight (resistance) or load to the movement as you get stronger.

Muscles Involved

Since this movement involves more than one major muscle group, it is referred to as a compound exercise. These three exercises work primarily the chest muscles. The secondary muscles that help with this movement are the anterior (front) deltoid (shoulder muscles), and the triceps (the three muscles located on the back of the upper arm responsible for extension of your elbow).

Technique

An important thing to learn here—and this applies to all exercises when you are gripping a bar—is your hand positioning. This is where most people get it wrong, and it is so crucially important. Rule of thumb is that when you place your hands on the bar—or handles, if you are in a machine—when you are performing the movement in and out, or off of your chest, your forearms should be moving straight up and down or in and out parallel to each other. If your forearms are pointed outward or slanted inward, adjust your hand position to make them parallel.

If you are using dumbbells or in a machine, lower the weight until you feel a good stretch across your chest, stop, and then press the weight out of that position by extending your arms until they are almost straight. With dumbbells, gradually converge the dumbbells as you are pressing up so that once you reach the upper position, the dumbbells touch together. You don't want to extend so far, though, that you place your elbows in a locked position. Stop just before the elbows lock. This is called keeping "soft elbows" and allows you to avoid injury to the elbow joint and also allows constant load on your triceps and chest; once you lock your elbows, your skeletal structure in your arms takes on the load, which removes the load from your muscles. So, constant load on the muscles involved is important throughout the entire set of ten to twelve repetitions.

If you are on a bench and using a bar, lower the bar with control until it touches (not bounces off) your chest, stop, and then push or press the weight back to the "soft elbow" position and repeat. Make sure you lower the weight to your chest with control. Go to www.gandmfitness.ca/startrightvideos to watch the videos.

SEATED ROW

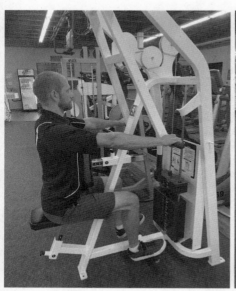
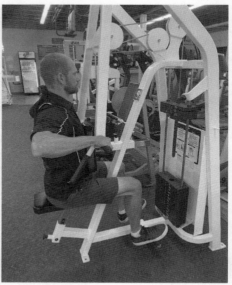
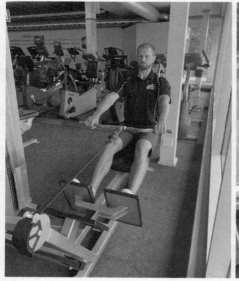
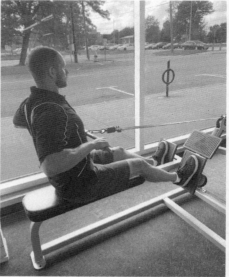

Introduction—Managing Risk of Joint Imbalance

Throughout your body, in order to keep proper balance of skeletal movement, there are antagonistic (opposing) muscle groups, muscles that work opposite to each other. When we are putting exercise routines together for clients, regardless of the client's goals, we must balance the exercise routine. In other words, we must take care that all antagonistic muscle groups are addressed in order to not create an imbalance in the skeletal joints.

For instance, I'm certain you've seen a sprinter go down in a race with a hamstring tear; it's a common occurrence. This typically occurs because the quadriceps (the four muscles in the front of the upper leg) of a sprinter are extremely strong and tend to overpower the hamstrings (the muscles in the back of the upper leg responsible for knee flexion and hip extension), so an imbalance occurs at the knee and hip joint, causing the weaker muscle group to be at risk of injury.

Shoulder joints are another example where joint imbalance is common. Most shoulder pain that I've come across with my clients is resolved once we correct the balance in the shoulder musculature. Usually the posterior (rear) deltoid (shoulder) muscle is very weak in comparison to the anterior (front) deltoid muscle and needs strengthening. Once balance is achieved, the pain is gone.

Some imbalances are very obvious just by looking at someone's posture. Many bodybuilders who aren't conscious of these possible imbalances typically have very strong and over-developed shoulder muscles in front from constant pressing movements and neglect to work the rear shoulder muscles. What this causes is rounding of the shoulders and palms turning backwards as they stand relaxed.

Muscles Involved

The risk described above is precisely why this rowing movement is next after the chest press. It works your upper body in exactly the opposite way from what the chest press does. You are pressing or pushing when you are working your chest, and now you will be pulling in order to address the opposite movement and the muscles involved, ensuring a correct balance in the upper body.

Technique

There are many different ways that you can do a rowing movement and several different variations, but here we will stick to the few basic movements.

You beginners will be using a seated, selectorized rowing machine to start—either the seated vertical row or what is usually referred to as the low row. Both are effective, and I still do them to this day myself. The only difference between the two machines is whether your upper body is supported by a chest pad. In the seated vertical row, you are seated with your chest against a pad. In the low row, you are also in a seated position, but you remain upright without the use or support of a chest pad. The seated vertical row eliminates the need to use your low back muscles to keep you upright, and the low row relies heavily on your low back muscles to maintain an upright posture throughout the movement. The choice is yours. You may want to start with the seated vertical row, and as your back gets stronger, you can advance to the low row.

The movements themselves are exactly the same regardless of which you choose. In both cases, you are in a seated upright position and holding perfect posture throughout the movement: chest out and up, with your upper body perfectly vertical to the floor. Grip the handles in such a way that when you are pulling, your forearms are parallel to each other, moving back and forth. If you are using the low row, there will be several bars and handles (accessories) to choose from. This is where most macho, would-be body builders get it all wrong. Your grip position, in order for this exercise to be as effective as possible, must allow you to retract your shoulders, with your elbows behind you. If you use a small handle where your hands are too close together, your hands will hit your body during the pulling back movement, thus limiting your range of motion and not allowing you to be able to get your arms back behind you to fully contract your back muscles for maximum effectiveness.

In both cases, grip the bar or handles with your palms facing downward, which will allow you to perform the movement with your elbows up. If you can picture it in your head, you will be mimicking the chest press movement but pulling rather than pushing. Again, work up to a resistance where you will reach muscle failure somewhere between ten and twelve repetitions. Go to www.gandmfitness.ca/startrightvideos to watch the videos.

SHOULDER PRESS

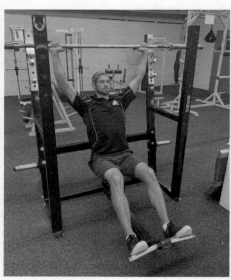
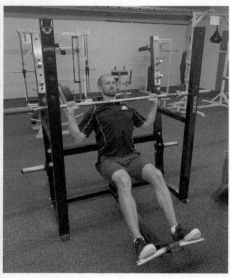
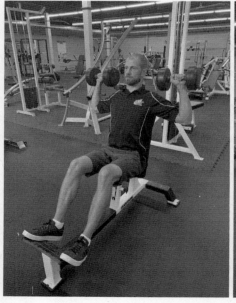
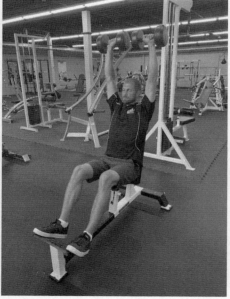

Introduction—Working the Middle Deltoids

These next two exercises—the shoulder press and the pull-down—are paired for balance, just like the seated row (above) is paired with the bench press, dumbbell press, and vertical chest press (above). They use opposite movements to ensure more balance in the upper body. The shoulder press is a pressing movement overhead; the pull-down is a very similar movement, but you are pulling down rather than pressing up.

Are you starting to understand the concept of balance and its relationship to pushing and pulling, and how it addresses opposing (antagonistic) muscle groups? If not, go back to the beginning of this chapter and reread. It's important because, sooner or later, you are going to want to change up your training routine, and you always need to keep this concept of balance in mind when doing so.

Muscles Involved

When performed properly, this exercise will isolate the medial (middle) deltoid (shoulder) muscle. Upright posture is key here in order to achieve that isolation of the medial deltoid. Leaning back will automatically shift the load to the anterior (front deltoid).

Technique

The shoulder press is a pressing movement where you start with your hand position at shoulder height and press or push the weight over your head until your arms are extended to the "soft elbow" position. You can perform this exercise seated in a machine, or you can use dumbbells in a seated position in a chair specifically made for shoulder pressing with a good, strong backrest and footrests to keep you in there nice and tight during the movement. You can also do this movement with an Olympic bar in a shoulder press bench specifically made for shoulder pressing with a bar (although I'm not a big fan of pressing with a bar). If you are not familiar with what an Olympic bar is, you will see one on pretty much every free weight pressing bench like the flat bench press, the incline bench press, the shoulder press, the squat rack, etc. where you would need to load the bar with the Olympic weight plates likely sitting on pegs on the sides of the benches or on a "weight tree" that is holding all of the weight plates.

So again, place your grip on the bar or on the handles of the machine where, when performing the movement, your forearms will be pointing and travelling straight up and down, vertical to the floor and parallel to each other. If your forearms are slanted inward or outward, adjust your hand position. If you choose to do this movement with dumbbells, it's all about balance and keeping your forearms under the weights as you press upwards.

If you are a beginner, I would suggest starting in a machine and then advancing to dumbbells once you have gained some strength, comfort with the movement, and confidence. If you are in a machine, the machine will dictate the path of the movement, so all you have to do is set the weight and make sure your hand position is correct. Push the weight up over your head to the "soft elbow" position and then lower the weight back down with control to the starting position without allowing the weight stack to bottom out, which would release the load from your shoulder muscles. You want to keep the load constant throughout the entire set of ten to twelve repetitions. If the weight stack bottoms out before you reach the bottom of the movement, the seat is likely set too low.

If you choose to go right to the dumbbell press, it's the same thing. Just make sure you are sitting up straight, never lean back or arch your back in order to lift the weight, and control the movement up and down. Using free weights like this is all about balance and comfort. Your forearms always need to be directly underneath the dumbbells when pressing out of the start position. You can press straight up and then down again, or you can gradually converge the path of the dumbbells as you press upwards so that the dumbbells actually touch together at the top position right above your head. Regardless of what position you want to end with at the top, converged or not, the path of the entire movement should always be in line with your body—not in front, not behind.

In the case of pressing with a bar (which, as I mentioned above, I'm not a big fan of), in order to perform the pressing movement, you are forced to arch your back and move your head back so you can lower the bar in front of your head in the bottom position prior to pressing up. As I had mentioned in the "Muscles Involved" section above, what this does is put the load more on the anterior (front) deltoid (shoulder) muscle rather than the medial (middle) deltoid, as a true shoulder movement is designed to do. That's why the seated position in a machine or with the use of dumbbells is a more effective way to work the shoulders: you are allowed to maintain a proper upright body position throughout the movement. Should you choose to use the bar for this exercise, do not do the movement behind your head. You'll see a lot of old-school lifters doing this, but it is not necessary, and it certainly places a lot of unnecessary stress on your neck. Furthermore, there is no advantage to lowering the bar down behind your head as opposed to in front. Go to www.gandmfitness.ca/startrightvideos to watch the videos.

PULL-DOWN

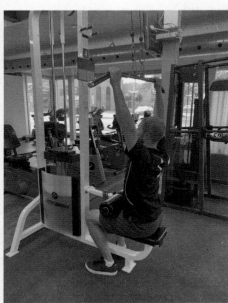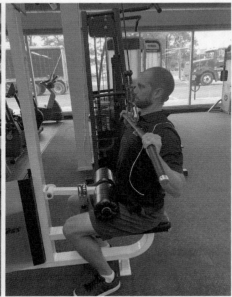

Introduction—Balancing Opposing Muscle Groups

This movement is the exact opposite of the shoulder press (above). Rather than pushing the weight up from shoulder height to an extended arm position above your head, start this one with an extended arm position above your head, and pull down against a load to shoulder height.

Muscles Involved

The muscles that make this movement of the rotation of the scapula possible (the scapula is the flat triangle shaped bone on each side of the spine in your upper back), is the latissimus dorsi muscles or "lats" which attach your upper arms to the mid-section of your upper back. They are the muscles that form the "v" shape in your back.

Technique

There are a few important things to learn here that most people are not aware of. The first is your body position. Be seated with your legs secured under the pads so you are being held down while completing the movement. If the pads were not there, you would eventually get to a point where the weight you were trying to pull down would pull you out of your seat, so you have to be anchored down. Once you slide your legs under the pads, you need to sit up straight with good posture and hold that body position throughout the movement. Where most go wrong is as the weight resistance starts to get more challenging, people tend to lean back to make it easier to pull the weight down. If you do lean back, you essentially turn this exercise into a rowing movement rather than a pull-down. The only thing you'll have to do in a good upright body position in order to complete this movement properly, if you are using a bar attachment, is to arch your back a bit and move your head back to avoid hitting the top of your head with the bar. Some machines have split handles so you don't even have to do that.

Do not pull the bar down behind your head. This is another thing you will usually see from the old-timers who don't realize that it is much safer, more comfortable, and just as effective to pull down in front of your head. You certainly don't want to pull down behind your head if you have a ponytail behind you. We've had to rescue several women and some guys also, when the clasp that attaches the bar to the cable catches their hair and nearly hangs them.

The other thing that is extremely important with this exercise is your hand positioning. As I've mentioned before, a rule of thumb is that with the proper hand position, you should see your forearms moving straight up and down. The forearms should not be slanted inward or outward. The reason people don't place their hands in the correct position is that they assume that you place your hands at the end of the bar, on the bends at the end of the bar, or on the rubber grips. That's not correct. Everyone has different shoulder widths and arm lengths, both of which will determine where your hands should be, rather than the length of the bar or where the rubber grips are on a handle. You need to suit yourself and your own body size. Stick with the rule of thumb and place your hands where they need to be regardless of what the bar or handles look like.

So, place your hands where they need to be on the bar or handles prior to sitting down. Once you have a grip, sit down and place your legs underneath the pads, sit up straight with good posture, and hold that position. Pull the bar or handles down until your elbows are at your side. This is the bottom of the movement and where you stop. This is also where most people make a mistake by pulling down too far. The only way to pull the bar down further than where I described is to turn your forearms forward, and that's wrong. Your forearms should stay pointing straight up and down throughout the movement. Once your hands are just below your chin, forearms still straight up and down, you are done pulling down. Now let the bar back up to the starting position (arms extended above your head), with control. Always control the weight on the way back. Repeat until you reach muscle failure between ten and twelve repetitions. Once you are done your set, stand up, let the weight stack gently set back down to release the load, and then let go of the bar or handles. You are done. Go to www.gandmfitness.ca/startrightvideos to watch the video.

BICEP CURLS

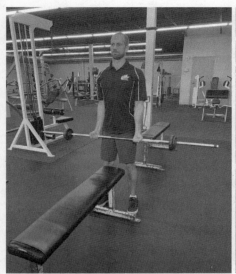
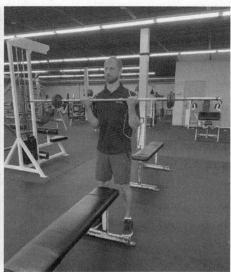
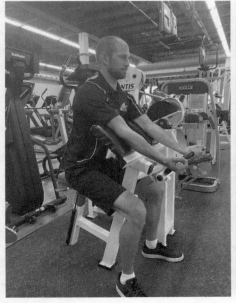
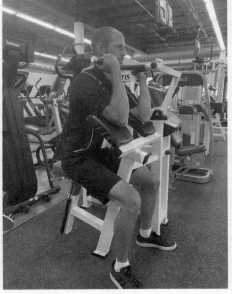

Introduction—Bending the Elbow

There are so many variations of this exercise, it is exhausting—there are standing barbell curls, standing dumbbell curls, seated dumbbell curls, preacher curls, spider curls, hammer curls, reverse curls, incline curls, Scott curls, and many more. For the purposes of this book, we will stick with the basic movement.

Muscles Involved

The bicep curl does one thing. It makes your bicep muscles, which are located on the front of the arm just above the elbow, shorten to flex or bend your arm at the elbow joint. Remember that.

Technique

This is a one-joint movement and does not involve any other joint, so no matter what variation of this exercise you do, the object is to keep your upper arm in one position. Your upper arm doesn't move or change position ever throughout the movement, no matter which exercise you do. If it does, you are not performing the exercise properly, or you are cheating. When you keep your upper arm still, you are only using the biceps to move the weight, nothing else. That's what we are after. So, focus, because as the resistance gets more challenging—whether it be from using more weight or being at the end of your set, doing the last few more challenging repetitions—your body will intuitively want to move your upper arm or change your body position in order to help you curl that weight without even realizing it. You need to really focus on your form.

As a side note, generally speaking, your body will do things for you automatically without you even realizing it is happening. It has many defense mechanisms that are naturally built in to protect you from injury. As I stated above, once you learn the proper technique (of any exercise, for that matter), you still need to focus on your form, even once you've been doing the same exercise for years like me, because your body will always try to do what it needs to in order to lift a weight the easiest way possible—and that's to recruit other muscle groups to assist in the movement.

So, with that in mind, we will start with the standing barbell curl—or, if you want to start in a machine, the seated bicep curl machine. In our gym we have a seated bicep curl machine that mimics seated dumbbell curls. If you can't find one of those in your gym, you'll likely be using a seated preacher curl machine, which has a slanted surface or pads that you rest your upper arms on to stabilize them while you are curling the weight.

If you choose to start with the standing barbell curl, stand with the loaded or pre-loaded bar in front of you on the end of a flat bench. Some gyms (like ours) have pre-loaded bars that are all welded up with the weight plates on the ends of the bar and weigh a certain amount. They usually go up in five pound increments so you can choose the one you want without having to load plates on the ends of the bar yourself like on the Olympic bars. Don't be a dummy and put the bar on the floor. Place the bar on the end of a flat bench so you don't have to pick it up off the floor at the beginning of each set and place it back down on the floor at the end of each set. That's nonsense; it's silly and unnecessary, and now you know better. And since I've mentioned not placing the bar on the floor, let me tell you this. I've been training with extremely heavy free weights most of my adult life, and other than the one-arm row when you actually have to start with the dumbbell on the floor next to the flat bench, I've never let any of the weights I was using touch the floor, ever. In my prime, I would dumbbell press on a flat bench or incline bench with ninety-pound dumbbells, and even with that amount of weight, when I was done my set, I would sit up, stand up, and place the dumbbells right back on the dumbbell rack where I got them from. We'll demonstrate exactly how to sit up from a lying position with heavy dumbbells in the video linked to at the end of this chapter. If you plan on continuing with heavy dumbbell presses in your workouts, you should definitely learn how to sit up with heavy dumbbells rather than dropping them on the floor. Dumbbells and barbells should never be dropped on the floor, ever, in any gym, regardless of the environment. Most gyms will frown upon dropping free weights on the floor, so don't be the one who gets called out by the staff for dropping weights. Be respectful of the equipment and the facility at all times. Those who do drop weights on the floor just don't know any better, they don't know how to sit up with them, or they are doing it for attention and should read this book and watch the videos. Since you are reading this book and watching the videos, you won't ever be that person.

Anyway, back to the bicep curl. If you are in a machine, it's pretty simple because the machine will likely have a padded surface or pads of some kind to place your upper arms against to hold them in position while performing the movement. Here, all you have to do is curl the weight until you have collapsed your elbow joint and then carefully and with control move your arms to the extended position again. Keep "soft elbows" at the extended position to protect your elbow joint from hyper extending and risking injury. Repeat to muscle failure with a resistance that allows you to do ten to twelve repetitions properly.

If you choose to start with the standing barbell curl, it is up to you to hold your upper arm position at your side throughout the movement, as there will be no pads to keep them there. So, standing, grab the bar at the correct spacing with your palms facing upwards or forward. If you just stand there relaxed with your arms at your side, palms facing forward, that would be the correct natural placement of your grip on the bar, right where your hands would be at your side. Hold the upper arm position at your sides; stand up straight with good posture, chest out and up, feet apart; and then bend the elbow to curl the weight up to a completely collapsed position without allowing your upper arm to move backward or forward. Again, repeat to muscle failure between ten and twelve repetitions. When done, gently set the bar back down on the end of the flat bench. I said gently; do not drop it on the bench. If you drop a heavy bar on the end of a bench it may bend. Don't be that person. Respect the equipment. Go to www.gandmfitness.ca/startrightvideos to watch the videos.

TRICEP PRESS

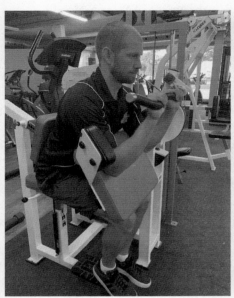
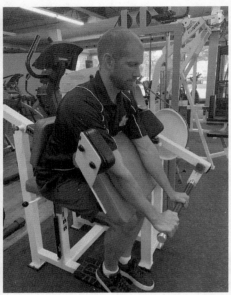

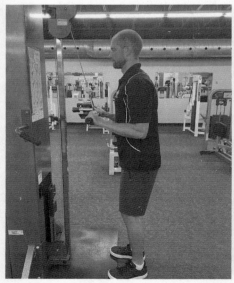
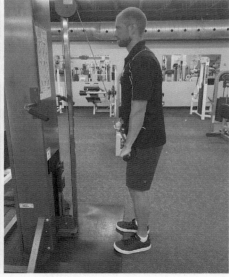

Introduction—Extending the Elbow

If you've been paying attention and are catching on to the concept of balance, you should have been able to predict that this exercise was next. If the bicep curl works to bend the elbow, then the tricep press should work to extend the elbow, and it does.

Muscles Involved

The biceps and triceps are opposing muscle groups. The three tricep muscles are located on the opposite side of the upper arm from the biceps.

Technique

Again, there are many different ways you can work this muscle group, but the way to start is in a tricep press machine or by a simple standing push-down movement done at a pull-down machine, one end of a cable crossover machine, on a duplex pulley machine, or anywhere where there is a cable hanging down from a high pulley with an available attachment that you can use specifically for tricep extensions. The tricep extension machine will look very similar to the curl machine, where you rest your upper arms on a slanted pad, except the handles will be at the top rather than at the bottom. Be seated with your upper arms resting on the angled pad, place your hands on the bar, and push down against the load without moving your arms off the pad or allowing them to slide up. This will ensure that you are isolating the triceps. Once you reach full extension of your arms at the bottom position, slowly let the bar come back up to the top, stopping before the weight stack bottoms out, which would release the load. We don't want that. Repeat down and up to muscle failure between ten and twelve repetitions. If you choose to use the pull-down machine or any of the other machines that have a hanging cable where you can place a tricep attachment, stand with your hand position at shoulder width on the attachment or bar, and, while keeping your upper arms at your sides, push down on the bar against the load until you reach full extension of your arms, and then slowly let the bar come back up with control until your forearms are just past parallel to the floor, while keeping your upper arms at your sides and not allowing the weight stack to bottom out. Repeat, and complete your set. Remember, there is nothing holding your upper arms still at your sides except you and your focus, so keep your form no matter how challenging the repetitions get toward the end of your set. Hold your form! Again, remember: "Your last heaviest rep of your last heaviest set should look no different than your first lightest rep of your first lightest set." Go to www.gandmfitness.ca/startrightvideos to watch the videos.

LEG PRESS

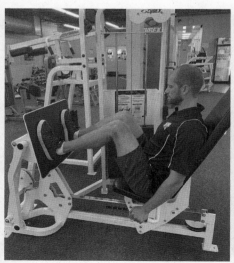 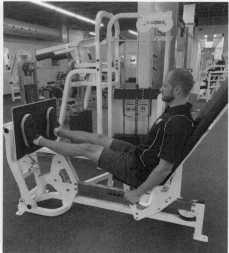

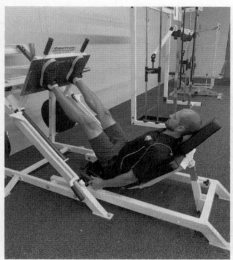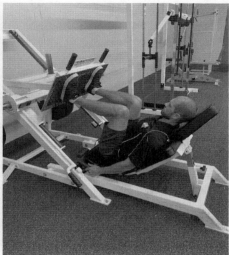

Introduction—A Compound Exercise

When you do an exercise that positions your body so that only one muscle group is able to lift a weight with no help from other muscle groups, you are essentially isolating one muscle group. Accordingly exercises such as the bicep curl and the tricep extension, are referred to as "isolation exercises." The leg press however, is not an isolation exercise, because in order to perform this movement under load, the body requires the work of two or more major muscle groups at the same time. As mentioned under "Bench Press, Dumbbell Press, and Vertical Chest Press," exercises such as these are referred to as "compound exercises."

Muscles Involved

When you perform a leg press, or a squat, the muscles groups used to complete these movements are the quadriceps (the four muscles located on the front of your upper leg responsible for knee extension and hip flexion), the hamstrings (the opposing muscle group located behind the upper leg responsible for knee flexion and hip extension), and the gluteus maximus, (butt muscles), also responsible for hip extension.

Technique

I chose the leg press exercise because it is the first step in a series of exercises that will eventually get you to perform a standing squat with confidence. You will likely find a leg press machine in every gym. There will be a plate-loaded version or one with a selectorized weight stack on the machine so you don't have to deal with loading and unloading the machine with weight plates. Regardless of the one you choose to use, the movement is identical. Be seated with your feet on the platform about shoulder width apart and high enough that you will remain flat-footed throughout the movement. If you place your feet too low, you will end up pushing with the balls of your feet; if your placement is too high, you'll find the pressure on your feet will be mostly on your heels. So, be flat-footed throughout the movement so the pressure on your feet will be felt on the entire foot. Push up or forward to lift the weight out of the resting position. If you are on a plate-loaded machine, you will need to move the resting hooks out of the way once you are holding the weight up in the extended leg position to allow the weight to come down past those stops. In the case of the seated selectorized machine, you'll likely have to move the seat up before you start as close as possible to the platform so you can just squeeze yourself in there, place your feet, and begin pushing. There are two things to keep in mind here, regardless of which apparatus you use. First, never allow your knee joint to "lock out" in the extended position. That will allow the load on the muscles to release and place the load through the knee joint. Don't let that happen. Keep a "soft" knee position at the fully extended position (knees just slightly bent). That will ensure that the load will remain on the muscles and not on the knee joint. Once at the top (leg extended position), let the weight down or back towards you until your knees are at or just past ninety degrees or square. You will know if you've lowered the weight too far if you feel your hips start to rotate upwards at the bottom of the movement and you feel a pulling in your low back. This is the second thing to keep in mind: your hips should remain still on the seat throughout the entire movement. Repeat as always to complete your set. Done. Go to www.gandmfitness.ca/startrightvideos to watch the videos.

ABDOMINAL CRUNCH

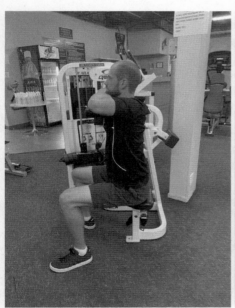
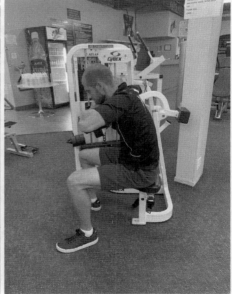

Introduction—Increasing Abdominal Strength

Believe me when I tell you that most people, whether beginners or seasoned veterans of weight training, haven't got a clue when it comes to training the abdominal muscles properly and effectively. Abdominal muscles should be trained no differently from any other muscle group, and yet, almost every day, I see people doing way too many repetitions and spending way too much time working their abdominal muscles. None of that is necessary.

Muscles Involved

Of course, when performed properly, any good abdominal exercise should isolate only the abdominal muscle wall including the oblique muscles located on the sides of the midsection of your body. There should be no involvement of any other muscle groups to help perform the movement.

Technique

Many, many moons ago, I was enlightened on the real, most effective methods to train abdominal muscles as I sat in a two-and-a-half-hour lecture on just that—how to effectively train abdominal muscles. The light sure went on, and I've been preaching this to my clients for over twenty-five years or more. There is far too much time and unnecessary effort devoted to abdominal training only because of lack of knowledge in this regard. The one thing that stuck in my mind and that was, to me, the most important message of the entire lecture was this: "The best way to most effectively work your abdominal muscles is to eliminate any and all leg involvement." Here's why. Recall what I wrote above about the difference between isolation exercises and compound exercises. True abdominal training should be performed as an isolation exercise, which requires you to eliminate the recruitment of any other muscle groups. Having said that, then, anchoring your legs or feet in any manner automatically recruits your leg muscles, and more specifically your hip flexors or quadriceps. Typically, people will place their feet under a couch if you are at home, or have a partner hold their feet down, or be in an abdominal machine that requires them to place their legs or their ankles behind pads. There are much more simple and effective ways, which I will describe here, to effectively train your abdominals without involving your legs at all. If you choose to start with a simple floor crunch, it doesn't get any easier than that. But here's where you need to understand exactly what it is you are supposed to do and what you are not supposed to do. You can choose to just lie on your back on the floor with your knees bent and your feet flat on the floor, or you can place a flat bench where your legs would be and rest your legs on top of the bench. You can also use your couch to rest your legs on if you are at home, if you don't have a flat bench handy. In both these positions, you have not anchored your legs in any way, so they will not be involved in the movement. So, that eliminates the first common mistake. Here, now, is where most people also get it wrong. Your abdominal wall covers the space between the bottom of your ribcage and your hips. The object here is to shorten that space, to bring your ribcage closer to your hips by curling your upper body forward, starting with your head and then your upper body, without allowing your low back to leave the floor at all. If you are lifting your lower back off of the floor, it is your hip flexors in your legs that make that happen, not your abdominal muscles, and in order for that to happen, you have to anchor your feet somehow.

Another thing: ideally, before you start, you should be in a pelvic tilt position, which is accomplished by tilting your hips so that you eliminate the natural space between your low back and the floor. Press your low back down so it feels the floor, and keep it there throughout the movement. Your arms will be at your sides to start. If you do your crunches in this manner, you will automatically stop the crunch where you should, because if you lift any further, your low back will leave the floor. Once you've reached that top position, reverse the crunch until you are lying flat on the floor again with your midsection completely extended. Repeat as many times as you can. If you find that you are doing too many and it is not a challenge, the way to make this crunch more challenging is to change the position of your arms. With arms positioned at your sides, you are not lifting the weight of your arms when you are crunching, so the next, more challenging position would be to cross your arms on your chest. Now, you will be adding the weight of your arms to the movement, making it more challenging. After that, the next, more challenging way to do the crunch would be by placing your hands behind your head, which moves the weight of your arms further away from your midsection, making it even more challenging. Don't pull on your head! You can also hold a weight on your chest. That'll certainly do the trick.

After that, you need an abdominal crunch machine so you can add resistance via a weight stack. Ideally, you will be looking for an abdominal crunch machine that does not anchor your legs or feet in any way. It will have a seat and a long pad at about chin height to rest your arms on. That's the best set-up. It will allow you to mimic a perfect floor crunch and the capability of choosing a weight from the weight stack that will get you to muscle failure between ten and twelve repetitions, just like any other exercise. The point here is that you train your abdominal muscles the same way as you train any other muscle group. For some reason, people think that you must do several hundred repetitions of crunches to be effective, which is incorrect. I'm certain that most people that are doing those hundreds of repetitions are convinced that they can reduce or eliminate the fat rolls around their waist by doing so. Nothing can be further from the truth.

You are looking to increase the strength of your abdominal muscles, and you know now how that is done: again, by using a resistance that will get you to muscle failure between ten and twelve repetitions, just like all of the other exercises you are doing; it's no different for abdominal training.

Once you find the machine, set the seat height fairly low, seat yourself, set the desired weight (start light), cross your arms, and place them on the pad in front of you. If you've set the seat low enough, you should be in a stretched upright position. Make sure you are in a seated position far enough forward that keeps you from bending at the hip. No bending at the hip! The crunch or bend should happen only at your midsection and nowhere else. If you are seated too far back, you will inevitably crunch down too far and end up bending at the hips. If you are performing this movement correctly, the only muscles that will be moving will be your abdominal muscles shortening and lengthening. That's it. And remember to not allow the weight stack to bottom out at the top of the movement. If it does this before you reach a good stretch in your midsection, then the seat is set too high. Go to www.gandmfitness.ca/startrightvideos to watch the video.

LOW BACK EXTENSION

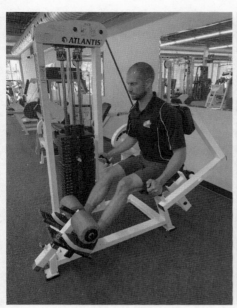
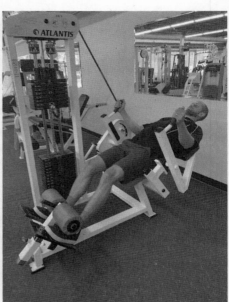
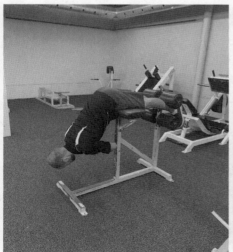
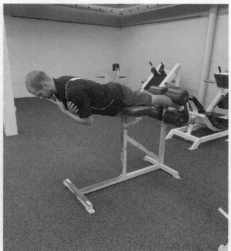

Introduction—Standing Up for Yourself

The muscle group that we are going to work in this exercise is responsible for keeping you upright when you are standing, thus making it one of the strongest muscle groups in your body. As long as you are standing, these muscles are working. These are your low back muscles. We treat these muscles a bit differently than all of the other muscle groups that I've discussed. We are going to train these muscles to keep them strong and functioning as they are meant to, so we will not be training them to muscle failure. That would take a lot of weight and effort and could result in injury.

Muscles Involved

Being located in your lower back area, these muscles are the opposing muscles to your abdominal muscles and collectively represent what everyone refers to as your core muscles.

Technique

Use a low back machine, which looks like a rocking chair, or a low back extension bench that you lay your hips on while hanging and facing the floor with the back of your ankles anchored behind some pads. Regardless of which you choose, the movement is the same. On the machine, choose a weight resistance using the weight stack; on the bench, the resistance will be provided by your upper body weight and increased by holding a weight against your chest. If you are using the machine in a seated position, you will rock back and forth as if you were in a rocking chair, except there will be resistance on your low back throughout the movement. Set the angle of the backrest so that you will be able to bend forward at the hips as much as possible under load, and then push back against the pad with your upper body until your body is in a straight, neutral position. Do not go so far back that you are arching your back. This is hyperextension of the low back, which is not necessary and should be avoided to prevent possible injury. Repeat ten to twelve times. Only increase the resistance when the set of ten to twelve repetitions is no longer challenging. If you are using the bench, the same rules apply. You will be "hanging" in the bottom position and then lifting your upper body up using your low back muscles and your gluteus maximus (butt) muscles, so that you end up in a straight, neutral body position at the top, facing the floor without arching your low back. Cross your arms on your chest while performing this one, whether you are holding a weight or not. If you have high blood pressure, do not do this one. You certainly don't want to be hanging upside down with high blood pressure. Use the machine, and avoid holding your breath while doing not only this exercise, but all exercises. Some deliberately use the "hanging" version because you involve the gluteus maximus (butt) muscles as you straighten your body, while the seated upright version eliminates the use of those muscles. Go to www.gandmfitness.ca/startrightvideos to watch the videos.

THAT'S A WRAP

So, that's it for the basic exercises. Do them all in one workout. Perform one light set as a specific warm-up, and then do two or three heavy sets to muscle failure. This basic workout should take you no longer than forty-five minutes or so. Take at least one or two days between workouts for adequate recuperation, and then repeat. The cardio component of your training (see chapter 20) can be done every day, and probably should be.

IT'S ALL GOOD

You now have all of the information and knowledge that you need to walk into any gym, join with confidence, and start your training with no assistance from anyone. You may be a bit nervous at first, but what you need to understand is that this chapter is meant to teach you the most effective ways of performing those exercises. Whether you do them perfectly or not, the most important thing is that you are doing them. As we say in our strength training seminar, "It's all good!" Whether you are doing the exercises perfectly or not, there is benefit from just "doing". Every workout will feel better and look better with practice. Just give yourself some time because practice makes perfect.

In the remaining chapters, you will learn about other aspects of your training that will help you get the most out of your time at the gym, so read on when you are ready.

NOTES

CHAPTER 11:
Frequency and Duration

Now that we've gone over the basic exercises that you will start with (see chapter 10), there is much more to learn in regard to getting the best results from your efforts.

CLASSIC OVERTRAINING—MORE IS NOT BETTER, UNLESS IT'S MORE REST

Most people think that if they are getting a certain result from doing something or consuming something—that if they do more or take more—it will be even better. Not so with strength training. Let me explain why.

In the simplest terms that I can use, your body will adapt to almost any situation you throw at it. It is meant to survive, so that's what it does. It adapts to survive or cope. In regard to strength training, most think that you gain the benefit or strength when you are training, and that can't be further from the truth. The truth is, you benefit while you are resting. This is when your body is over the stress of lifting against a load and is finding a way to adapt—to better cope with the stress if it happens again—and that's when your muscles rebuild and get stronger. You actually break down muscle tissue when you are lifting against a load, and rebuilding better, stronger muscle when you are resting.

So, you should recognize the importance of proper rest. If you are not resting enough, you will inevitably be overtraining, and that will backfire on you sooner or later. You'll get tired more quickly, get injured, get sick, or even stop seeing results, simply because you are not allowing your body to recover and adapt sufficiently.

During those fifteen years when I was competing in amateur bodybuilding, I often befriended others at the competitions who were doing the same and were very successful at it. Those were the guys I'd ask advice from. Lo and behold, the one I asked the most advice from advised me, right off the bat, to take an extra day off for rest during the week for better results. Go figure.

Therefore, if you are just starting out, you will stick with the basic exercises and do them every other day, or better yet, every third day—certainly not every day. Training the same muscle groups on consecutive days is classic overtraining by someone who doesn't know better—and now, we all know better, right?

Once you get confident and stronger, you will find that you want to do more exercises for a particular muscle group, but if you keep adding exercises to your basic routine, it will end up taking way too much time to complete. The solution for you when you get to that point is to break up your routine; rather than train all of the major muscle groups in one workout, you will "split" your routine into fewer muscle groups each workout. That way, if you train only three muscle groups in one workout, and the others in another workout, you can train on consecutive days because you are not training the same muscle groups in those two workouts. This type of split would be referred to as a "two-day split."

Perhaps in the first workout you would train your chest, your back, and your biceps. Then, in the second workout, you would train your legs, your shoulders, and your triceps. Add your calves and abdominals to whichever workouts you want—or, better yet, create a short, third workout just to work your calves and abdominals. That would serve as an additional rest day for your upper body. Good idea!

The idea of splitting your workouts will continue as you get more confident, more experienced, and stronger. There are three-day splits, four-day splits, five-, and six-. What you have to keep in mind is getting adequate rest days. A rule of thumb would be to take at least one or two full rest days from lifting weights after three consecutive days of weight training.

Another thing about overtraining: I've been in my club and watched members work out very hard for up to two straight hours or more. Wow, that's another perfect example of classic overtraining. If you recall, in chapters 8 and 10 I mentioned how the human body has many natural defense mechanisms built in to protect us from injury. Here's another. There is a stress hormone called cortisol that gets excreted throughout your body when you are under stress, all kinds of stress, including mental and also physical stress from lifting heavy weights. Research shows that once you've trained with heavy weights for about fifty minutes or so, cortisol shows up to act as a buffer to ensure that you won't or can't build muscles that your natural body can't handle. So, if you are killing yourself for over an hour because you still believe that more is better, you are wasting your time. You'll get more benefit by going home and resting. So, no matter how many body parts you are training and how many sets you want to do, always keep in mind when constructing your weight training workouts that you should be done lifting in less than an hour. Be confident that if you are lifting to muscle failure, focusing on your strict form, and giving one hundred percent each and every workout, that one hour or less is all you will ever need. Trust me.

NOTES

CHAPTER 12:
Weight, Reps, and Sets

Now that we've covered frequency and duration of your training routine and rest (see chapter 11), let's talk about weight, repetitions, and sets. Typically, we recommend, as I've mentioned numerous times already, ten to twelve repetitions per set to muscle failure. That's the safest and most effective way to gain strength as a beginner. That will change a bit as you get more experienced, stronger, and more confident. As a beginner, always choose a very light weight to start with on your first set. This will serve as a practice and warm-up set and gives you an opportunity to better assess what weight to choose from there. It is better to gradually increase the weight until you find what resistance you'd like to start with that's not too challenging at first. Better that than choosing a weight that is too heavy and finding out in the middle of your set that it's too heavy. Also, you can't judge whether or not it is the right weight by how the first few repetitions feel. It's the last few that count. I've come across this many times while training people. They do one or two repetitions and then stop and proceed to tell me that they think it's too light. Take my advice and just do the entire set; then judge. Most of those people ended up eating their words by the end of the set.

No one can tell you what weight you should start with because everyone has different strengths in different parts of their bodies, and only you can determine, by trial, where to begin. So, be careful, and don't be a hero. Although I've been weight training myself for over forty years, I still do a warm-up set of each exercise I do. Sometimes several light sets. It better prepares me for the real heavy stuff. So, even though I may be able to dumbbell press with ninety-pound dumbbells, you will often see me pressing with the thirty-fives, the forty-fives, and the sixty-fives before heading closer to the real heavy ones. Doing things in that manner has kept me pretty much injury-free over all these years. In the end, the weight that you will work with is the weight that will bring you to muscle failure somewhere between ten and twelve repetitions. Do three to four sets to start: a light warm-up set to better prepare the muscles involved for that particular movement, and then three heavy sets with the weight you've found previously that will get you to that muscle failure between ten and twelve repetitions. Those weights will change as you get stronger. Eventually, the weight you were failing with between ten and twelve repetitions, you will suddenly find, as a nice surprise, you are able to do fourteen repetitions of. This means it's time to go heavier; if you don't continue to use heavier weights once you are over the twelve repetition mark, and you find yourself lifting that weight fourteen, fifteen, sixteen times or more, you will not get any stronger. By continuing to use that weight for that many repetitions, you are now training for muscular endurance rather than strength training. It's why strength training is commonly referred to as "progressive weight resistance training." That's how it should be treated: as a progression in weight resistance resulting in progressively stronger muscles. Remember what we learned in chapters 8 and 11 about the body adapting to its environment and stresses? If you continue to use the same weight resistance that you are quite capable of lifting many, many times without a challenge, then your body has nothing to adapt to, as the ability and level of strength required to lift that weight are already there. Get it? Good.

NOTES

CHAPTER 13:
The Importance of Negative Contractions

This is by far the one thing where I feel the most people go wrong in their workouts and miss out on a tremendous amount of gains, simply because they don't know what a negative contraction is and how it benefits those looking to increase their strength as efficiently and effectively as possible. All muscles have the ability to contract (shorten) and extend (lengthen) in order to create movement of the skeletal structure. It's the importance of the lengthening phase that so many seem to not realize and thus not perform properly or deliberately. It's unfortunate, because this phase of the lift is extremely beneficial and helps tremendously in building strength.

What's even more unfortunate is that most of the people I see not emphasizing the negative contraction are the veteran lifters. Most people think that once you've lifted the weight you're done. They lift it slowly and with purpose and then drop the weight back to the starting position with no effort to slow the return or negative phase down. As I wrote in chapter 7, there are two phases to every lift: the positive (shortening) of the muscle group and the negative (lengthening) of the muscle. A simple example that illustrates this perfectly is the bicep curl. Assuming you are starting at the extended (straight–arm) position, when you bend the elbow to curl or lift the weight, the bicep shortens to enable that to happen. That shortening of the biceps is the positive contraction. In order for you to let the weight back down to the start position again, that same muscle group has to lengthen in order to result in an extended or straight-arm position again. That's the negative contraction of the biceps, and in my mind, is as important as the positive or lifting of the weight, if not even more important. Remember this one thing, and you'll never neglect the negative phase of any exercise again: "Negative contractions build strength."

Imagine what those veteran lifters who are not aware of the benefit and don't put any effort into the negative contraction are losing out on; every set, every exercise, every workout, every day, every week, every month, sometimes for years. What a shame. But now you know better. When I am in my club and I hear weights hitting the floor harder than I would like, or a weight stack on a machine slamming back down at the end of someone's set, I get upset. I post signs all over the gym about dropping the weights. Most people think that it just has to do with abusing the equipment and the facility (and it does somewhat), but it has more to do with the absence of gain from not doing the negative contraction. Unfortunately, most don't realize the latter. But now, you do.

Picture yourself on a seated leg press. You perform with perfect form nine repetitions, and you are at the top (extended) leg position, and you know you won't be able to do another press. Now you know to bring the stops in and slowly bring the weight down until it rests on the stops. That's how it's done. So, when you see someone else on the leg press and hear the "bang" at the end of each of their sets, you will then think and feel exactly what I think and feel when I hear it.

I'll offer here a few more points about the negative contraction that you should be aware of that most aren't. One might think that if you can't do another repetition, and you are at muscle failure, how can you bring the weight back down slowly and with control—not only on the leg press, but for any exercise? The answer is simple. You are much stronger on the negative contraction than the positive contraction; although you are not able to physically do another repetition or lift, you can certainly do another negative phase without much effort at all, so do it every time and reap the benefit. And keep in mind that there is a negative contraction in every repetition you do, so control, control, control, lifting and lowering. The more emphasis you put on the negative, the more benefit (strength) you will gain from the exercise.

Lastly, before we put this subject to bed, I'm going to share with you something that most, if not all veteran lifters and bodybuilders do not know or are not aware of. A lot of times, you'll see veteran lifters training with a partner, which is a great idea. Partners help keep you motivated and help with the lifting when needed. So, here's my point: let's take the bench press, for example. The person doing the pressing does his or her nine, ten repetitions and starts having a hard time, so the partner standing at the head of the bench now acts as the "spotter." The spotter helps his or her partner perform a few more repetitions at the end of the set, repetitions that the lifter would not have been able to do without the spotter's help. But one thing, if you watch closely: the spotter needs to help with only the lifting phase, but no help is required to help the lifter bring the bar back down to his or her chest slowly and with control, and now you know why. The thing that most veteran lifters don't realize is that the spotter is not there to help the lifter do more repetitions; rather, they are there to help the lifter do more *negatives*! Consider yourself schooled.

NOTES

CHAPTER 14:
Progression

The technical term for strength training is actually "progressive weight resistance," the most important of those words
being "progressive." If you recall (and you should, because I've
mentioned it several times now) how our bodies adapt to what
we do to it—whether it is malnutrition, physical abuse, mental
abuse, sleep deprivation, or whatever—if we are challenging
ourselves when strength training, lifting to muscle failure,
and getting enough rest, we should progress and get stronger.
Think of it this way, keeping the adaptation concept in mind:
if you use the same weight resistance every time you do a
certain exercise, for the same number of repetitions, over and
over again, what is it that your body has to adapt to? "Nothing"
is the answer. On the other hand, if you do your first set as
a specific warm-up, increase the weight resistance for the
second set so you are reaching muscle failure at about twelve
repetitions, increasing the load again for the third set so you
are reaching muscle failure at about ten repetitions, and then
a final set with again more resistance, reaching muscle failure
at eight or nine repetitions, you will definitely see strength
gains. What will happen is eventually (and it won't take that
long), the weight load you were using for that second set
will become your new warm-up weight, the weight you were

using for the third set where you were failing at ten repetitions you will now be able to lift for twelve repetitions rather than ten, and the weight you were using in your fourth set where you were failing at eight or nine repetitions you will now be strong enough to lift ten times or more. Therefore you will add another set with a brand new weight, more than you were capable of lifting before, because you have forced your body to adapt to the challenge and create more strength in the muscles involved in that movement. Granted, some of the gain at first will come from your body getting used to the movement, but once you are comfortable and your body is more familiar with the movement, the rest is nothing but strength gain.

So, that's how you progress. It's not the number of repetitions that is important. It could be twelve, ten, nine, or even eight. The most important thing is that you perform each set to muscle failure, and the rest will happen naturally. You will get to a point where you will reach a plateau and have a very hard time increasing the weight any more. That's only natural. In that case, as long as you are still lifting to muscle failure, you will maintain the high level of strength that you have achieved. Be proud of it, and don't take it for granted.

In today's world of electronics and gadgetry, our lives have become "easy." What I mean is that most, if not all, of the physical exertion that was required of us thirty, forty, fifty years ago or more is no longer required, as more and more gadgets and machinery are invented to keep us on our behinds longer than we should be, doing nothing more than pushing buttons. Accordingly, strength training, which used to be considered an optional elective or recreational activity, is now a mandatory part of all of our lives, and it's because of the lack of physical exertion that is making us all weaker than we should be, no matter what age we are. So consider yourself weaker than you should be, and do something about it.

NOTES

CHAPTER 15:
Consistency

If I were asked what I thought would be the single most mis-understood concept concerning exercise success—the concept that would be of most benefit, if understood, to those aiming to get into shape, stronger, and more flexible in the most effec-tive, efficient way possible—I would have to say consistency.

I've come to this conclusion from watching others and also from personal experience. I, too, was one of those young, eager guys, with more energy than I needed and an attention span of a two-year-old. I'd go from one thing to another—whatever interested me the most at the time—and thus, although one of my favourite pastimes was weightlifting, I often got side-tracked by other interests. That was quite normal for someone my age at the time, but looking back now, I recall working out for three months and then stopping for a month or so when something distracted me that I felt should get my full atten-tion; then returning to the gym again for several months, just to stop again for a while until I felt it was time to return—over and over again for several of my first years working out. The gains I made at that time, training off and on like that, were still good, and I could see the difference, likely because of my age and the plentiful supply of testosterone and growth hormone naturally present in my body. But I realize now that if I had been more consistent, the gains would have been substantially more significant. But such is life, and now I'm able to tell you about it so you don't fall into the same bad habit as I did.

You need to keep in mind that this new habit of working out at your local gym must be a lifelong commitment, so treat it as a job, and just do it. Do it consistently and with commitment, regardless of the distractions that life will throw at you along the way. It's that important. Again, coming from personal experience, I was and still am the worst at consistency because of my nature. If I can't give something 100 percent, I tend to not do it at all, and that's been an issue for me all of my life. Those distractions I mentioned—whether a personal problem, a work issue, or any issue, for that matter that weighed heavily on my mind—would keep me from the gym. Just being upset about something would be enough to sabotage my progress and keep me home. Silly, I know, but that's me. So, don't let that be you. Get to the gym and do your workout, regardless of where your mind is. It's certainly better to do a half-assed workout than to not do one at all. Just commit to putting that one hour aside for nothing more than taking care of you and nothing else. We have a saying in our seminars that sums this up, short and sweet: "Stop stopping." I should take my own advice.

I'll make one more point here to hammer home this topic of consistency and how important it is. Once again, from personal experience: if I couldn't get to the gym often enough to complete my three-day split or four-day split that week, I felt like I was wasting my time and was training for nothing, always trying to catch up and make up for lost time, so I would quit for a while, frustrated, until I convinced myself that I should go back. Well, I'd like to tell you about a customer that we have at our gym that will drive home this point of consistency because it is the perfect example of how consistency trumps everything else. We'll call him Fred. Fred joined us about seven years ago. He was a very busy financial advisor who sat on his behind most of the day. Fortunately for him, was aware of the health risks associated with that type of a job. He was approaching retirement age and smart enough that he knew what he had to do. When he joined, he told us right away that he could commit to only one day a week, but that he would not miss that one day. He promised. My son has been training Fred for seven years now, consistently one day a week without fail, and the gains, although they could have come more quickly if he trained more often, still did come. He just recently retired and is in great physical condition, by leaps and bounds more physically fit than when he first walked into our club. Now, if he had my mentality, he would not have joined at all; but he did, he made the commitment, he stuck to it, and he's now very happy that he did. Once a week!

So, don't think that if you miss a few workouts here and there, you are not getting anywhere, and end up stopping out of frustration. Just resume when you can, and keep looking ahead. You'll be glad you did. So, now you get it. Commit and stay committed.

Another point about consistency is that once you've committed and have been at it for quite some time, you will begin to take for granted the improvement in your physical self. It happens all of the time. You tend to forget how out of shape you were at one time, and, as time goes by, your new physical condition, although very good, seems to feel just normal. The only way that I've observed a person would realize that they are taking their new physical condition for granted is when something happens that keeps them from exercising, like a health condition or injury. Then, and only then, do they realize, when they finally return to the gym, how good a physical state they were in prior to having to stop exercising, because everything seems heavier, harder, and more of a challenge than ever. I've heard dozens of times in our gym, when people experience this kind of break from their regular exercise routine, "It's like starting over!" It only takes approximately seventy-two hours for the level of fitness you've achieved to start to diminish if you are not able to continue your workouts for one reason or another. Although your progress may not be as quick as you would like, the decline of your fitness level will certainly be quicker than you would expect. "Use it or lose it!"

So, now that I've revealed to you one of my weaknesses as a young lifter, I'd like to close this chapter by redeeming myself, and tell you about something I did that illustrates first-hand what real commitment can do. One day, at the age of about twenty-one or so, I looked down at my legs and thought, "I'd really like to build some very strong and muscular legs." I knew at that time that most young lifters hated training their legs and focused all of their time at the gym on the upper body. In my mind, those individuals looked silly. It was obvious. They had big, strong, muscular upper bodies and what I would refer to as "table legs." I wasn't about to let that happen to me, so I made the commitment to train my legs consistently for as long as it took to build the muscular legs that I was after. Fast forward ten years—yes, ten years of consistent, heavy training, rarely missing a leg workout, even when I was sick. Have a look at the picture on the next page. Those are my legs at fifty-two years of age! I trained them consistently for years, but only once a week, and using only one exercise: squats—perfectly performed squats. I knew full well that when I stepped on stage in all of those bodybuilding competitions, my legs would keep me in the top three every time, and they did. And back then, in the late nineties, it was commonplace to have twelve to sixteen competitors in one weight class, so finishing in the top three every time was an accomplishment, for sure. Also, competing against the "cheaters" and finishing in the top three was an acknowledgement of how hard work and consistency would pay off. The gains I made in the amateur bodybuilding phase of my life were made with good, old-fashioned hard work and consistency—no drugs, stimulants, or anything else. Some may argue to the contrary, but I just look at that as a compliment. If there are those out there that think I've built my physique with drugs, then kudos to me, because I didn't. I was and still am a "lifetime natural amateur body builder" and will always remain such.

So, there you have it. If you are not convinced by now that consistency is of utmost importance, you haven't been paying attention—so, go back and reread this chapter!

NOTES

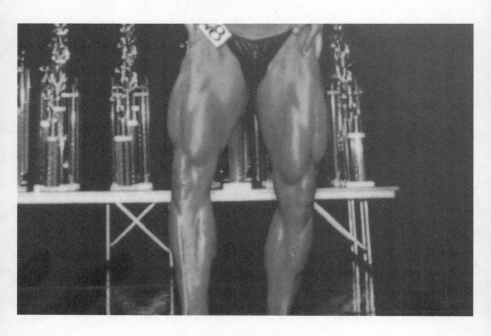

Picture of my legs.

CHAPTER 16:
Focus

I've touched on this earlier in the book, but it's so important that it deserves its own chapter. No matter what you do in life—for work, pastime, or sport—without focus, results suffer. That's the bottom line. Our worst enemy when performing work, sport, or even everyday things like driving a motor vehicle is distraction. The world is full of distractions that grab our attention, and more often than not, the distractions are a disruption of focus. We must then deliberately zone out and ignore them if we want to get the most from our efforts in life.

Strength training is no different. The distractions in a gym environment are plentiful—from friends wanting to "shoot the breeze" with you, to the member that takes a liking to you and won't stop asking you questions, to—and let's face it, this is the truth—scantily dressed gym members, to music, phone texts, magazines, and so on. These are all distractions and need to be eliminated or ignored or avoided at all costs if you really want to get the best results from your training. Do you think a butcher handling a knife sharp enough to sever a finger effortlessly is talking to a friend by speaker on his iPhone, or singing along with his favourite song on the radio, or thinking about what he's going to do or where he's going to go after work? No. If he wants the best result possible from his efforts, he will focus on what he is doing and end up with beautifully cut meat and still have all of his fingers when he is done.

Driving is another great example. If you are reading this and old enough to drive, you know as well as I do that just talking to someone while driving is a distraction—let's face it. So, I'm going to use myself again as an example of how true, deliberate focus can reap the best results possible. If you recall the effort I put forth when I decided to build up my leg muscles (see chapter 15), you may remember that I first decided and made the commitment to myself that I would train my legs once a week, very hard, and never miss a workout unless I was gravely ill—and I didn't. I trained very hard, I was consistent by training once a week for years without missing a workout, but that was only a part of the reason I made such great gains in my leg musculature.

The other important component that was required to build those legs was laser-sharp focus during my leg workout. Here's exactly what I did, each and every leg workout for years. It all started first thing in the morning. I would wake up and literally think, "It's leg day!" Not, "It's Friday," or, "It's Sunday," or "It's Valentine's Day," or, "It's my birthday." Nope—"It's leg day." Even if I still had to put in a full day at work in the factory before I could get to my leg workout, all day long, to me, it was "leg day." That's how important my leg workout was to me. Once I got to the gym, I did everything I could to avoid distractions. This sometimes became a problem. Some members on the floor working out at the same time as I was would think that I was being anti-social because I wouldn't stop and talk to anyone. I actually tried to avoid eye contact. After a while, that changed because those members who saw what I was doing on that one day a week, week after week, began to realize that it was "leg day" for Gino. Don't talk to Gino.

I would start by sitting on an upright bike in the cardio area and riding the bike for about ten minutes. This would be the first part of my warm-up to ensure adequate blood flow in my leg muscles and joints. After that, I would head to the squat rack. I'd set up a flat bench so I could be sitting and facing the squat rack between sets, not facing the rest of the gym and the other members. I would place my knee wraps, my water, and my weight belt on the flat bench beside me. The knee wraps and belt I used only on the last few, very heavy sets for some extra support and to help avoid injury. Then, I would do some stretching. I'd stretch right there in front of the squat rack for a few minutes, stretching not only my legs but all of the major muscle groups in my body. That was the end of my preparation prior to beginning the actual squats. Then it was time to do some specific warm-up sets, and they were many. I did this on purpose to give my body, and especially my legs and leg joints, plenty of time to prepare for the heavy sets to come—again, to avoid risk of injury. All of this preparation prior to performing the heavy squats certainly paid off because I have never had to deal with any kind of injury to my back, my knees, or my leg muscles, ever.

And before I get into what I actually did for my leg workout, keep this in mind because it also speaks to how focused I was with every repetition and every set that I performed. My squats were performed with perfect form, each and every repetition, without fail. Each rep was slow and deliberate, thinking about nothing other than how it felt in my legs. Perfect form and laser focus every second of every repetition of every set. In between sets, I would sit on that flat bench, facing the squat rack, thinking of nothing other than preparing my mind and my legs for the next set. I would not allow my mind to wander.

First, I would perform a set with only the Olympic bar on my shoulders, just to get my body to perform the movement and be better prepared to do it again with more resistance. The Olympic bar weighed in at forty-five pounds. Another set followed with the bar and a forty-five-pound plate on each end (one hundred and thirty-five pounds), then another set with the bar, the forty-five, and a twenty-five on each end (one hundred and eighty-five pounds), then another set with the forty-five and a thirty-five (two- hundred and five pounds), and then another set with the bar and two forty-five-pound plates on each end. That last set would be a total of two-hundred and twenty-five pounds, and still to me was considered a warm-up set. Now it was time to move on to the more challenging sets. I would add a ten-pound plate and a five-pound plate to each side, bringing the total weight to two-hundred and fifty-five pounds, and I performed usually about twelve repetitions with that weight. Then I took the ten and five off and replaced them with a twenty-five-pound plate on each side, which brought the weight up to two hundred and seventy-five pounds. I would be able to perform at least ten to twelve perfect repetitions still with that. Then I removed the twenty-five-pound plates from each end of the bar and replaced them with thirty-five-pound plates, bringing the total weight to two hundred and ninety-five pounds. I would usually be able to get at least eight to ten repetitions with that weight. Next, I replaced the thirty-five-pound plates with forty-five-pound plates, so there were three forty-five-pound plates on each end of that Olympic bar, bringing the total weight to three hundred and fifteen pounds. This was when I usually started wrapping my knees and using the belt. I could usually perform six to eight perfect repetitions at that weight, with no help, no spotter, just me and my laser focus. If I was having a good day and I was able to do at least eight reps with that weight, I would perform a "bonus" set with three hundred and thirty-five pounds. I'd usually do three or four repetitions only with that weight, but those three or four repetitions were still done with perfect form. Once I was done with that, I stripped off all of the plates and returned them to their proper place, packed up my stuff, and went home.

Yes, believe it or not, that's all I did for my leg workout, and that's all I needed. And for that matter, if you focus as much as I did, that's all you will need too. When I was done, I felt like someone beat my legs to a pulp with a bat, and I could barely walk properly. I repeated that same routine each and every week, without fail, for many years, and that's how I built those legs in the picture. No drugs, no stimulants—nothing but good, old-fashioned focus, consistency, and very hard work. Today, at sixty years of age, I can still look down at my legs and smile because that muscle is still there and I'm very proud of that accomplishment to this day. There are many, many twenty-year-olds that wish they had a set of leg muscles like mine. Many of them could not believe that I did only squats and nothing else. They would often ask why I wouldn't consider doing lunges or something like that after my squats to finish off. My reply would always be this: "If you are doing your squats properly and enough of them, you should not be able to walk properly, let alone do lunges afterwards. You should be falling on your face if you tried to." That would give them something to think about.

Funny thing—a few years ago, as I got older and the heavy squats were starting to take their toll, in order to maintain that muscle mass in my legs without doing heavy, free-weight squats any longer, I switched to the leg press. Same thing, though. I do those leg presses with laser focus, commitment, and perfect form. The funny thing is that my legs are so strong that I fill the entire leg press machine with forty-five-pound plates! Usually nine of them on each side of the machine! I can tell you that you get a lot of looks from others in the gym when you are pressing that much weight, especially in a gym where no one knows you. No one expects a one-hundred-and-ninety pound, sixty-year-old member to be pressing almost half a ton for six to eight perfect repetitions. The hardest part of my leg routine now is loading and unloading all of those forty-five pound Olympic plates. So, if you ask me if I think I would have achieved the same results if I had let distractions sidetrack my focus, I would have to say no.

NOTES

CHAPTER 17:
A Few Words about Advanced Exercises and Techniques

At first thought, my initial intentions were to write a chapter like this in a prominent position, listing and describing advanced exercises that some of you might be interested in doing once the time comes to introduce more of a challenge to your workouts.

After some serious thought, I've come to remind myself that this book is not primarily about advanced workouts. This book is mainly for the beginner—the young, eager, energetic adolescent who wants to start getting in better shape—and for anyone else, senior or otherwise, who is just looking to join a gym for the first time without knowledge or experience.

Rather than place advanced information in the middle of this book, information that's perhaps not for every reader, I decided to add it all to the end as bonus chapter 1. It is there to read when you are ready, when you are more familiar with weight training exercises and techniques and interested in taking your fitness to another level. Or, don't read it at all if you are not interested.

Furthermore, there are several ways to increase the challenge in your workouts using the same exercises. You don't have to change your exercises. You can do the same exercises but in a different way or order. You can slow the movements down to increase the intensity through the movement, or you can shuffle the order of your exercises, or both! So, to that end, I will give what I feel is the best advice I can if and when you feel that you'd like to at least investigate the possibility of introducing more advanced exercises into your routine.

Here's my best advice: Hire a trainer. Hire a good one, too. You get what you pay for. The so-called trainer with very little experience, very little education in the health and recreation field, and a matchbook-cover certification that certifies a person with an open-book, online exam is not the person you want to hire. If you are thinking about price, well, yeah, it's going to be a bit expensive, but "expensive" is a relative term that depends on what you are comparing it to. I'll just ask this: What is your health worth to you? It's not an expense. You can't look at it that way. It's essentially an investment in your health and education.

So, when it's the right time for you, and you've read bonus chapter 1, if you decide to go the personal trainer route, you don't need to hire them as a babysitter, unless you really need to be accountable to someone to keep you going. You just need to hire the trainer to do a consultation and assessment, come up with a new program design, and teach it to you. Once that's done, you shouldn't need them anymore. I'm confident that the routine that your trainer will come up with will consist of most if not all of the advanced exercises that are described in bonus chapter 1.

At our gym, we have one price that includes all of that, so you get it all in one shot—one time, done. You'll get the assessment/consultation, the new program, and the training in the gym. The information you will get from us or any good trainer will serve you in the gym for many, many more months of training and outside the gym for a lifetime, and is worth every penny. As I said, and I'll say it again, "It's not an expense. You can't look at it that way. It's essentially an investment in your health and education." Enough said.

NOTES

CHAPTER 18:
More Cool Tips That Make a Big Difference

When one has trained with weights for as long as I have, trained in multiple gyms as I have, watched other professionals as much as I have, and trained as many people as I have, you gain a special kind of experience that not many others have. I've seen the best and the worst. I've seen the best (others like myself) and the worst—those fresh out of school that do what the books tell them to do—and a lot of them are graduates of a Kinesiology program with very little experience lifting weights themselves, so they just don't have the hands-on experience in regard to how a movement should really feel because they haven't experienced it themselves long enough. It's sometimes as new to them as it is to their client, which is unfortunate for the client. As such, though, you learn as you do.

In my case, the more and more I lifted those weights and studied over the many years, the more I learned and was made aware of all of the little idiosyncrasies and small adjustments in your body positioning and technique that make a big difference. I've made these kinds of suggestions and corrections hundreds of times to seasoned veterans in the gym, and most were very surprised at how such little changes could make such a big difference.

Here are a few examples of how a little tiny change makes a big difference.

"RULES OF THUMB"

Pull-downs or chins are a good example. When you place your hands in the anatomically correct position on the bar—which we've previously discussed (see chapter 10), so you should know by now where that is—most will just naturally grab the bar by wrapping their hand around the bar with their four fingers over the bar and their thumb under the bar, and that works. It's natural to grip that way. Here's the change: Why leave your thumb under the bar where it is not contributing to any of the pulling? Place your thumb over the bar along with your other fingers so you are now adding the thumb as an extra gripping tool to help you more easily hold onto the bar longer and pull with more force. This helps because some people will stop the repetitions before they get to muscle failure because they can't hang on to the bar any longer. This happens a lot with heavy shrugs also: your hands give out before your muscles doing the movement do. If you have turned yourself into a serious lifter, the addition of wrist straps along with placing your thumb with your other fingers can make a huge difference in your gripping ability.

The same thing is true when you are pushing against a handle or bar. If you are not a seasoned veteran, I would not suggest this with a free-weight Olympic bar because it's a bit risky, but if you are in a machine, veteran or not, place your thumb under or alongside your other fingers. This will ultimately create for you an extra pad to rest the bar against when you are pushing against it, so the pressure of the handle will not dig into the palm of your hand as much as if your thumb were placed on the opposite side of the bar. Try it—you'll like it, and it'll help, once you get used to it.

BUILT-IN CARDIO

Here's another one. Try not to take any more time between sets than you have to. A rule of thumb, in my opinion, would be no more than one minute. Try it. You'll be surprised at how short a time that really is, if you are working hard and training each set, like you should be, to muscle failure!

I realize that this one can be a challenge, especially in an atmosphere like we have in our club. Everyone is extremely friendly, and sometimes I think that in a lot of cases, people are there more for the social aspect of seeing their friends than getting the best workout for their money. That's okay with me too, so whatever floats your boat—and as long as you are happy in our club, it's okay with me. Companionship, camaraderie, good friendships, and good conversation with those you look forward to seeing three or four times a week somewhere at a mutually convenient gathering place like our gym is certainly a huge benefit to anyone's general health and well-being. So, be your own person, and do what works for you.

This is one of those suggestions that make a difference without having to change any of the exercises that you are doing. It adds a cardio component to your workout without having to step on a cardio machine at all.

DON'T HOLD YOUR BREATH

Next, don't hold your breath, ever, while doing your repetitions, especially the last few hard ones. This is important. If you have high blood pressure especially, you never want to hold your breath while lifting. This will skyrocket your blood pressure temporarily while you are pushing that resistance, which could cause issues that could be life-threatening, so always breathe out while doing the lifting part of the move-ment (the positive contraction), and then take a nice, deep breath in while lowering the weight back to the starting posi-tion (the negative contraction) to expand your diaphragm again with fresh air. Generally speaking, everyone should be breathing like this during every lift because you don't want your tight, inflated diaphragm to help lift the weight; you just want your muscles to do it on their own. So, don't hold your breath. Always breathe out on exertion.

KEEP THAT LOAD ON

Here's another tip we mention every time we train someone on how to use a machine, but it's worth repeating. Never let the load release between reps. By that I mean you need to set the seat or chest pad or whatever adjustments can be made to suit your stature, to ensure that when you are bringing the weight back down to the start position, the weight stack does not set back down, which would release the load from your muscles between every repetition. The load must be consis-tently maintained throughout the entire set of repetitions to get the most benefit. So, if you hear the weights banging or touching between each repetition, stop and do whatever adjustments are needed to avoid letting that happen.

With the more advanced exercises, locking of the joints is probably one of the biggest issues, as doing that also releases load from the muscle group being trained and detracts very much from the potential gain from that set of repetitions— saying nothing of the risk of possible injury to your joints. So, think about the consistent load on the muscles you are using while doing your set, rather than looking around to see what everyone else is up to while you are doing it. Focus.

ANCHOR YOURSELF

This tip is extremely simple but also extremely beneficial. I have been doing this all along and still do it today. When you first start training with free weights, safety should be top of mind, and we will touch on that subject later on in bonus chapter 1. One of the things that helps protect you from possible injury when you are doing any lying presses, or pullovers on a flat bench with free weights, is to place your feet on the floor to anchor yourself side to side and prevent you from falling off the bench. If and when you have done those free-weight exercises for a while with your feet anchored to the floor, try doing those exercises with your feet on the end of the bench rather than on the floor. What that will do for you is force you to balance your body side to side on the bench by using your core muscles—more specifically, your obliques—as stabilizers, rather than your legs. Whether I'm doing flat or incline dumbbell presses, or head cavers, or dumbbell flys, or any free-weight bench exercises, my feet are never on the floor; they're always on the bench. What this new body position will also do for you is place your low back in a more neutral position and keep you from arching your back too much, which happens a lot when you're struggling with the heavier weights with your feet on the floor. Good one!

DON'T BE REDUNDANT

One last tip. This concerns the choice of exercises. This is one that I see a lot of veteran lifters doing incorrectly. If you are creating your own program and trying to choose what exercises to do, keep in mind that the exercises you choose to do may be redundant. What I mean by redundant is that simply changing a hand position or a foot position doesn't necessarily mean that you are doing anything differently, as far as the muscle you are training is concerned. A perfect example is the tricep extension. Let's assume that you are putting together a split routine and are able to choose three tricep exercises for the routine. You choose standing tricep extensions with a bar; then the same extensions, only with a rope to change the hand position from palms facing the floor to a hammer grip on the rope; then one-arm extensions on the same machine. These are all redundant exercises. Why? Because in order to work the tricep muscles differently with each exercise, you need to change the position of your upper arm in relation to your body, not change the hand position. So, my choices would be close-grip presses first, which would place your upper arms out in front of you; then dips, which would place your upper arms behind you; then standing pushdowns or extensions, which would place your upper arms in line with your body. That's how it's done.

The same thing applies to bicep curls. Standing and doing bar curls, then dumbbells curls, then reverse curls will only change the action of the forearm muscles, not the biceps, so they are again redundant. You would choose a standing bar curl, which would place the upper arm at your sides; then a preacher curl, which would place your upper arms in front of you; then, lastly, some incline dumbbell curls, which would place your upper arms behind you. Get it?

There are many, many more of these tips that I've learned, but most of the remainder are directed at the seasoned veteran, so I won't go into those here—but if you hire that experienced trainer that I described earlier, when you are ready for the more advanced exercises, you'll likely learn a lot of them, especially if you hire me!

So, as you can see, there are plenty of things that you can do to get the most out of your workouts without even changing the exercises, but only if you are aware of them. Consider yourself now part of the few that are aware. You now have the information advantage.

NOTES

CHAPTER 19:
Range of Motion

The range of motion of a particular movement refers to the ability of that particular limb or body part to move at the primary joint from one extreme or limit to the opposite. For example, moving your lower arm from a completely extended position (straight arm) to a fully collapsed position (fully bent) is the range of motion of the elbow joint. As I've alluded to several times in this book, although working to full range of motion is important, once a load is placed on any particular body part, it is prudent to pay attention to and be aware that sometimes it is not safe to take the motion to the extreme ends of the range. Remember the "soft elbow" reference when doing an exercise like the preacher curl so as not to overextend the elbow, and avoiding the "lockout" position of a joint like the knee joint when doing leg presses. Protecting joints like these by not fully extending is correct and should help avoid any risk of injury to that joint. It's better to be safe than sorry, particularly in strength training, as a joint injury will certainly set you back in your progress. So, always use full range of motion, but avoid full extension or hyperextension and any lockout position of the joint involved.

You may be asking yourself why using the full range of motion is so important. Well, in a nutshell, here's the answer. Remember this statement:

You build strength in only the range of motion that you move.

So, having said that, here's what typically happens when I correct someone that is not travelling in a full range of motion and then tries to do so. A perfect example is the squat. In the squat exercise, the proper range of motion would be to start at a standing position with soft knees. That would be the top of the range. The bottom of the range should be when you reach a point where your thighs are parallel to the floor. By doing a squat that way, you are travelling through the full range of motion properly and safely.

Typically, as the weight resistance gets heavier, the natural response by your body is to not go down to the bottom of the range, so as the weights get heavier and heavier, the range gets shorter and shorter, turning a perfect squat into what is referred to as a half-squat.

Many times in my own gym, I've overheard a member boasting about how much weight they can squat. Well, not to brag, but I can pretty much tell by just looking at someone that what they claim they can lift is likely not true, or it is true in their minds only because they don't realize that they are not doing the exercise the way it should be done. When the opportunity presents itself and I get the chance to actually watch them doing their squats, I'm usually right; they are doing half-squats, even quarter-squats, but certainly not full squats.

Here's the problem that presents itself almost every time. When someone neglects to use the full range of motion while doing the heavier sets of squats, and then gets corrected by someone like me, the typical response is to correct the range without lightening up on the weight, so they get stuck at the bottom and cannot push themselves out of the full squat position. Why? Because, and let's say it together:

"You build strength in only the range of motion that
you move!"

So, going down into the bottom position is still doable because that's the negative contraction, and we all know now that you are much stronger on the negative contraction than the positive contraction. Furthermore, all of that weight on your shoulders certainly helps to get you down there. But once that person is down "in the hole," as I refer to it, it is extremely difficult and sometimes impossible to launch out of that bottom position because there is not enough strength built up down there to get back up. Get it?

I also see this frequently on the bench press. As the weight gets heavier and heavier, the range gets shorter and shorter. With the lighter load, the person brings the bar down to just tap his or her chest and then lifts, but as the weight gets heavier and heavier, the bar seems to get further and further away from the chest. And once that gets corrected, and the lifter does not lighten up on the weight, we know now what happens. The weight will come down to the chest as it should, but it won't go back up "out of the hole," and we all know why.

The other point that needs to be made here about why training to the full range of motion is so important is that if you constantly use a shortened range of motion, this practice will inevitably result in a lack of flexibility. When strength training, your muscles have a tendency to want to shorten as you continually contract your muscles under load—so always, always, always use the full range of motion properly and safely for the best results.

NOTES

CHAPTER 20:
Cardio

This is a simple concept, at first thought, but there is surprisingly much to explain and much to learn about this effective kind of training. First of all, it does not build muscle size, but, if you want to be at your physical best, regardless of the fact that you may be in the gym to build muscle and strength, cardiovascular fitness will still contribute greatly to your results. Here's why, in a nutshell: effective cardiovascular training increases efficient blood flow to all areas of your body. The more efficiently that happens, the better and more effective your training will be, and the results will come faster. It's far too technical for our purposes here to get into the medical explanations and descriptions of how and why that is, so you'll just have to trust that I know what I'm talking about. All you need to know is that the more efficiently your cardiovascular system can carry fresh, oxygenated blood around your body, the better in all respects.

CARDIO FOR HEALTHY BODY FAT LEVEL OR ENDURANCE

Cardiovascular training can be performed with two results in mind: weight loss or enhanced cardiovascular fitness for long-term endurance like running, rowing, or any sport where you need endurance. Training is done differently for each desired result. The difference will be where your heart rate is during this training. If you are looking to control or lose your body fat, you will be trying to maintain a constant heart rate of between sixty-five and eighty-five percent of your maximum heart rate the entire time you are doing your cardio training, preferably closer to the sixty-five percent. The answer to the questions "when" and "for how long" are: "after your strength training, not before" and "for at least twenty minutes." There is a direct correlation—proven by science, not me—between where your heart rate is maintained and how much body fat will be used during your cardio training. It's slow and steady for fat burning, and higher intensity for athletic endurance.

I'll try to explain here, and not make it too technical, why doing your cardio after strength training, not before, is so important if you are looking to reduce or maintain a healthy body fat level. Your body has three energy systems available to it. The first one, and the one that's used up the quickest, is cellular energy referred to as ATP (Adenosine Triphosphate). This type of energy store comes directly from your muscle cells and is there for immediate, maximum, and short-term effort like a short sprint. It doesn't last more than about ten seconds at full exertion when your heart rate is at its maximum. That would be the only time this type of energy is recruited. The second source of energy comes from the glycogen stored in your muscles that is created from the food that you eat. This energy system will last you at least twenty minutes or much longer, depending on how much effort you are putting into your strength training, or any training, for that matter. But that energy source will also run out eventually. The third energy source that will take over from there, but really doesn't want to, is your fat stores. So, it should make sense to you now that if you deplete the first two energy systems available to you while you are doing your strength training routine and then do your cardio at the end, you should be using fat stores for the energy you are going to need to get you through your cardio. If you do your cardio first, you likely will not be using any body fat, as the other two energy systems will be available to get you through it. Get it? So, cardio training comes at the end.

Now, back to the heart rate part. As mentioned above, you can do cardio training for fat loss, maintaining your body fat level, or you can train for endurance. If you are training for endurance, you can do this training anytime, but you must maintain a heart rate of over eighty-five percent of your maximum heart rate. You'll be breathing heavily, but as your cardiovascular system becomes more efficient with time, you'll become more comfortable and be able to maintain it longer. You can do either type of cardio training as often as you wish.

I'm sure by now you are asking how to determine what your heart rate should be in those ranges I just gave you. It's simple mathematics. Use this general guideline: For fat loss or fat control, use two hundred and twenty beats per minute to start the calculation, as this is approximately your maximum heart rate as a newborn. You lose approximately one beat every year of your life, so at age fifty, it would make sense for you to have a maximum heart rate of approximately one hundred and seventy (220 − 50 = 170). If you do some simple math, you should find that the range for this type of fat control or fat loss training at age fifty should be maintained at somewhere between one hundred ten and one hundred forty-four beats per minute. That would represent sixty-five to eighty-five percent of your maximum heart rate. In this range, you should be able to still carry on a conversation without getting out of breath.

If you are training for cardiovascular endurance, your heart rate should be kept above eighty-five percent of your maximum heart rate.

These concepts have been debated for many years; many professors and lecturers are convinced that a calorie is a calorie, and that just burning calories, no matter how you do it, is just as effective for losing body fat. I strongly and respectfully disagree. I say, follow what the fitness experts and fitness researchers say, not the professors that preach their opinions from a desktop. I've done it many times myself, preparing for bodybuilding contests by using the advice of the fitness professionals, and it works each and every time, just the way it should. Doing cardio how and when you should and eating properly are the keys to success in this department.

So, who are you going to believe—someone who's done it successfully many times over and successfully trained others to do the same, or one who teaches it from the information that is given to them in their studies and has never done it themselves? Take your pick.

CARDIO MACHINES

One more question that is often asked about cardio training is, "What cardio machine do I use?" Here's my advice: It depends on what fitness level you are at when you first start. Although I'm a big advocate of challenging yourself (as you should be aware of by now), if your fitness level is poor, you have to use common sense here. Start with a bike, recumbent or upright, so you are seated and comfortable. You can safely gain cardiovascular fitness gradually there, and then, when you feel it is time, you can graduate to a standing activity like the treadmill.

Even though you can do a really good cardio workout on a treadmill if you use the incline and position your body properly, people tend to be lazy on the treadmill and do not get the workout they should. So, once you've mastered the treadmill, I would suggest moving on to another cardio machine like an elliptical trainer that mimics running without any impact on your joints. Once you feel you have achieved a more advanced level of cardiovascular fitness, try my favourite, the stair climber. If you are younger and have more energy than you need, get right to it and jump on the stair climber. No sense in waiting—get to it.

One last little bit of advice about doing cardio. If you are doing it standing up, like on a treadmill, stair climber, or elliptical, listen closely to these next three words, and always follow this advice:

Stand up straight!

The bars and handles located on these machines are there for balance—not to hang on to for dear life. The typical mistake people make on the treadmill is that when they decide to crank up the incline to get a better workout, they grab onto the console and hang on—so, essentially, they end up leaning back with the incline and holding on to the console so they don't fall off the end of the treadmill. To correct this mistake, just keep one thing in mind: your body should always be vertical or perpendicular to the floor no matter how high the incline is set. Imagine yourself climbing a steep hill. You have nothing to hold on to, so you lean forward, not backward, in order to hold your body position straight up and down in relation to a flat surface. So when on the treadmill, if you are doing it correctly, you should be able to let go of the side rails and still hold your position, regardless of where the incline is set.

The stair climber is the same. The side rails are there for balance, not to lean on. I've seen people actually lock their arms and hold themselves up while on the stair climber to make it easier to do the movement. They are essentially removing some of their body weight from the steps by holding themselves up. Once you are accustomed to using the stair climber and comfortable, you should be able to not hold on to the rails at all. Another thing I notice that happens a lot on the stair climber is very small steps. Some people barely bend their knees at all; they just move their ankles. Making sure that you get at least a six- to eight-inch stepping movement will ensure that your quadriceps and gluteals get the workout they should.

The issue using the elliptical is also the leaning forward on the rails. Stand up straight, and keep good posture always.

These simple little suggestions will allow you to get the most out of the use of these machines—and that's what you want, so don't cheat! You are only cheating yourself out of additional gains by not doing it properly.

I think I've touched on most of the pertinent points here concerning cardiovascular training, so enjoy!

NOTES

CHAPTER 21:
A Few Words about Nutrition

Boy, I could write an entire book on the subject of this chapter ... and, oh, I actually did!

If you are not already aware of it, I self-published my very first book back in 2012. It's called *Eat Smart, Eat Often, Eat Small* ("The S.O.S. Book"). All of the advice I've ever given to anyone asking about how, when, and what to eat is in this great little book. Easy to read and understand, it has helped hundreds of our members and outsiders alike to learn to eat properly, using good, old-fashioned common sense, to achieve their optimal body weight. It teaches the reader that if you make better food choices, eat more often during the day, and eat in the correct amounts, your excess body fat will melt away like butter on hot bread.

The information in this book is based on science and personal experience both, and I haven't seen these recommendations fail anyone yet. It hasn't failed and won't because it corrects the most common mistakes people make when it comes to eating habits—more specifically, bad eating habits—that inevitably cause our bodies to store excess body fat. The three simple rules in this book have been used by bodybuilders for decades and still are today because they work. I've often said that if you happen to be at a bodybuilding contest, you'll notice right away that the spectators are generally overweight, drinking coffee and eating a muffin, but the competitors are underweight and eating highly nutritious food all day long. They carry their food with them all of the time (Eating Right) and eat approximately every two and a half hours (Eating Often) and in the correct amount (Eating Small). How about that! S.O.S.!

Eating the way this book describes makes your body function more efficiently, and as I say in the book, "With an efficiently running body automatically comes a reduction in body fat." It just happens because it has to. When you eat the way this book describes, your body has no reason to store excess body fat, none at all, so, *poof*—it's gone. I've competed in nine bodybuilding contests and used these principles religiously, and it worked one hundred percent of the time; not ninety, not eighty, but one hundred—each and every time.

You can also use the same principles to gain weight. It's science, and it works. I used it to gain weight for a strongman competition I did, and then used it again to lose the weight for a bodybuilding competition. Like I said, this is coming from personal experience. We offer the download of this book for free from our website, so go there and get it. You'll find it at www.gandmfitness.com. An avid reader can read through it in an hour and a half. This book will not tell you what to eat. It's based on calories in and calories out. Yes, you researchers and lecturers: calories in versus calories out—that's what I said. Researchers, professors, lecturers and the like—I've listened patiently and with respect to them all, and all I can say is that I've done it my way successfully every time, and they just talk about the way research implies that it should happen. Sorry for the harsh words, but that's the long and the short of it.

I truly am convinced by science and my own experience that if you feed your body good, wholesome, nutritious food as often as your body requires it and in the correct amount, you will reach and maintain your optimal body weight—no question. Eating this way not only will ensure that your body is constantly fueled properly throughout the day, but will help keep a healthy blood sugar level, which a lot of experts neglect to recognize as an important factor.

And here come some more harsh words. In my humble opinion, intermittent fasting is a joke. Deliberately starving yourself for a short period of time does nothing more than mess up your blood sugar. I've done intermittent fasting a lot in my adult life because I'm not a morning eater. I never have been. So, for most of my adult working life as a self-employed individual, I would eat my last meal of the day no later than seven thirty or so, and my first meal of the next day a lot of times wouldn't be until noon or one o'clock, sometimes even two o'clock, because I was so busy working away that I would lose track of time. Did it help me lose body fat? No. Did it give me more brain clarity as the researchers and fasting advocates claim? No. And can one really believe that eating nothing is better than eating good, wholesome, nutritious food? Consider this: When I worked in the factory from age eighteen to thirty-two, I ate breakfast at 7:00 a.m., ate again at the 9:30 a.m. break, ate again at lunchtime, ate again at the 2:30 p.m. break, ate supper after work at about 5:30 p.m., and then again at around 8:00 p.m. That's six meals. Did I gain weight eating that way? No. Was I able to maintain a healthy body fat level? Yes.

So, you decide. Eat good, wholesome, nutritious food often throughout the day and in the correct amount, or skip all those meals and just overeat whatever you can get your hands on when you are hungry, and see what happens.

And also, when these so-called experts suggest that people with serious, life-threatening health conditions like cancer consider long-term fasting, they are, in my humble opinion again, out of line, *way out of line.*

This craze of starving yourself to get your body to rebuild itself and discard the weak cells will pass, just like all of the rest of the bull advice going on in the nutrition industry, and we will all return to eating properly, often throughout the day, and in the correct amount. Research is just that—it's research and has to be taken with a grain of salt. More often than not, what is right today is often proven to be wrong tomorrow; something else then shows promise, and it starts all over again. So, if you want to do something extra besides your workouts to achieve that optimal body weight, do yourself a favour and read the book. I guarantee it will help. You're welcome.

NOTES

CHAPTER 22:
Final Words

I've spent most of my adult life hustling to make a buck any way I could, and I got pretty good at it. I had what seemed like endless energy, working a full-time job in a factory and at the same time running a health club, running a tanning supply company, making supply deliveries on the weekends, buying and selling tanning beds, refurbishing them, maintaining them for customers, working flea markets on Sundays with my in-laws, and so on. At the same time I helped my wife start a very successful dancewear business. I've run a small moving company, have flipped houses, acquired many rental properties spread all over southern Ontario, and now consider myself semi-retired. One of my good friends calls me a "serial entrepreneur."

Now that I am in the final quarter of my life, let's say, and I really don't have to hustle like that anymore, I find myself thinking more and more about giving back, paying things forward, like my knowledge of physical fitness, for instance. And that's exactly why I wrote this book. It's an opportunity for me to pass on what I've learned from being in the fitness industry over the past thirty-five years. I know it will help those who read it, just like I know my first book did. It would be a shame if I took all of this knowledge with me to my grave.

So, as I sat to write this final chapter in this book, I thought to myself, "What more can I pass on to these readers now, after spilling my guts out with pretty much everything I know about strength training and its benefits and the importance of joining a gym and its benefits?" I thought, and I thought, and I thought, and this is what I came up with. The decision to take up strength training is like any other decision you make on your own behalf, for your own benefit, in your lifetime. You make the decision to do something, and hopefully you follow through and benefit from that decision.

The big difference between the decision to take up regular exercise—more specifically, strength training in a gym—and all other decisions you will make in your lifetime is that the decision to take up strength training is (in my opinion) the smartest and possibly the most important decision one will ever make in their lifetime. It's that important. Here's the reason I say that: Although the reason most people take up regular exercise and join a gym is to help them lose some unwanted body fat, or feel better, or get out of the house, or in genuine concern for their health and well-being as they get older, the fact is that most if not all do not realize the enormous benefit to their general health and longevity that regular exercise offers. It's a scientifically proven fact, and all researchers in this field agree, for a change. You've essentially saved your own life.

One day at my club, as I was walking through as I normally would, simply to say hello to the members, I happened to notice one particular member riding a stationary bike, and I thought I'd stop and chat with him for a bit. This member just happens to be a medical doctor. His exact words to me in that conversation as we both looked around at everyone working out in the gym were these: "Gino, you guys are saving lives in here every day." All I could think of saying in response to that was, "I know," because I do know.

In my strength training seminar that I offer at my club, I often refer to gyms as "simulators." What a gym does for us now is re-introduce all of that challenging physical exertion that is missing from our lives and thus causing us to age and lose muscle mass and strength more quickly than we should. It seems very silly to me that we as humans will go to so much trouble and expense to purchase new technology that removes more and more the need for physical exertion, only to end up purchasing a gym membership to re-introduce it. Silly.

So, once you decide to join a gym, after you've found the one you prefer, join knowing that this decision to add exercise to your life is a lifelong commitment. Joining for a month or three months is ridiculous unless you are not certain that you will be comfortable in that particular gym and you need more time to try it out. The safest way to proceed with a membership is once you find the gym you want to join, join for a year on monthly payments. They will likely ask for banking information at that point, which is fine, now that you've made your decision to commit to that gym. This option will also be the cheapest. Should something go wrong and the gym closes, you simply contact your bank and stop payments on your monthly dues.

I hate to end this chapter with a "sad but true" story, but I feel that this one, a real-life example of what can happen to you if you let it, will drive home even more how important it is to seriously consider starting this exercise effort right away and commit to doing it religiously for the rest of your life. We have a member at our club that joined shortly after he retired. He explained to us that all of his working life, he slowly accumulated all of those "toys" that men typically acquire so they can have something to "play with" once they retire and have more time to simply "have fun" and "enjoy life." They'll typically have a mobile home parked in the driveway, boats, four-wheelers, sports cars; they have scuba gear, skis, hockey equipment, and the like. Well, fast forward to this person's retirement, and lo and behold, because this person was the typical "work until you retire and then enjoy your toys" kind of a guy, he found himself in such bad physical condition that he was forced to sell all of his toys because he just "couldn't enjoy using them." He was physically not able to use them. What a shame. Don't let that be you. Don't let your physical condition be an afterthought. It should be top of mind always, each and every day of your life.

NOTES

CONCLUSION

So, we have come to the end. My hope, now that you've read the entire book, is that you now have a better understanding of how and why it is so important to join a health club, strength train, and make your regular visits there a part of your life for as long as you live.

If you haven't joined a health club before, my hope also is that you are now more comfortable, confident, and eager to actually go join that club.

As I mentioned in the Introduction, I've been strength training now for over forty years. I started when I was sixteen, and I'm now sixty, so do the math: that's forty-four years. As a result, to this day, at sixty years of age, I can't think of anything that I could do physically as a teenager that I can't do now. As a matter of fact, I'm stronger now than I was then.

As we age, without strength training, our posture will inevitably be negatively affected, and we won't carry ourselves as upright and confident as we once did. It's because our back muscles are not keeping our shoulders back where they belong, resulting in a rounded back and a slouched, slightly leaned-forward look. That's a shame. Don't be that person. There are certainly things that we can't control as we age, but some things we can control, and keeping good posture is one of them. Let strength training keep you standing up straight with confidence and a bounce in your step for as long as humanly possible.

In my humble opinion, a generally healthy individual should never be burdened with the thought of not being able to physically do something until very late in their lives. The inability to physically perform a task from adolescence to over eighty should never enter your mind if you do what you should to take care of your physical self properly, consistently, and safely. The most recent research in strength training proves that.

If you are a young adolescent, you have a great head start over most and are a smart cookie for realizing at such a young age that strength training is an integral part of living a great life. Middle-aged or senior, trust me when I tell you that if this is something you've never done before, it will change your life.

Strong, confident, and vibrant is how everyone should look and feel, whether an adolescent, middle-aged, or a senior—at least in my mind. It's all about the quality of your life, and that, my friends, is all up to you and how you choose to live your life. And remember, it's never too late.

Yours in good health,
Gino A. Spada

BONUS CHAPTER 1:
Advanced Exercises

Oh, boy—I'm so excited to be able to offer this chapter because this is what I live for. I consider myself an advanced lifter, and I do these advanced exercises all of the time and have been for years. The following exercises are my favourites. They are mostly compound exercises and what I feel are the most effective ones in regard to strength and muscle growth.

THE DANGERS OF HEAVY WEIGHTLIFTING

Just like any other exercises that I've described earlier, you need to learn how to do them properly in order to get the most and intended benefit from them. As the heading states, they can be dangerous if you are not careful. I'll be offering a video of them at the end of each description as I did with the basic exercises (see chapter 10), so there will be no excuse for doing them incorrectly. Read the description, and then watch the video. I know that even the most seasoned veteran will learn a lot from this chapter alone.

MY LEAST FAVOURITE EXERCISES

At the end of this chapter, because I'm assuming that if you are reading this chapter you are the ones most interested in gaining lots of strength and muscle mass, I will also list a few of my least favourite exercises with an explanation of why they are my least favourite and why I recommend that you just stay away from them. In my professional opinion, if you are working out primarily to increase your muscle mass, they are a complete waste of time and effort.

SPOTTING

As an added bonus, I'll explain in depth what a good spotter should know how to do and when. Sooner or later, you will end up with a partner, and a good partner must be a good spotter; otherwise, he or she will be nothing more than a cheerleader.

This is a huge chapter with loads of great information, so focus! Let's start with the exercises.

DIPS

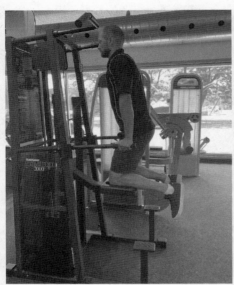
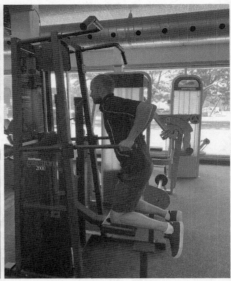

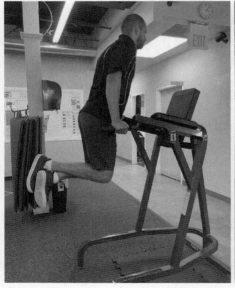
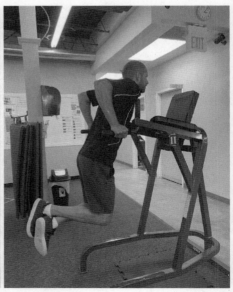

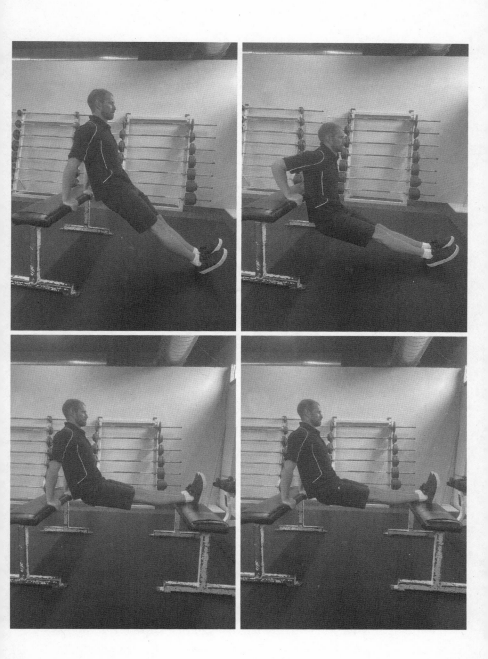

Introduction

As I have mentioned several times previously, and is worth mentioning again here, is, if you are focused on building muscle mass, there are two things that you should always keep in mind when deciding which exercises to incorporate into your workouts. One: only choose exercises that you can lift heavy weights with, and two: choose compound exercises whenever possible.

Muscles Involved

This exercise is primarily meant to build the triceps, but, as most don't realize, there are many other major muscle groups that are also under a tremendous amount of load when you are doing this one—namely, the trapezius, the pectorals, and the deltoids. It pretty much works your entire upper body, similar to the push-up.

Technique

If your gym does not have a Gravitron or similar machine, this one's going to be difficult right off the bat because the resistance you are forced to use will be your entire body weight. If that's the case, do them anyway. You may only be able to do one or two, or maybe three, but it's a start, and if you keep at it, you'll be doing ten or twelve in no time. Trust me, it's worth the effort. Once you've reached that point, the way to increase the load is to use a belt made specifically for this movement. It looks like a weightlifting belt, but it has a chain attached. This special belt will allow you to hang a weight from the chain. If your gym has a Gravitron, as ours does, this machine works the opposite of all of the other machines with a weight stack on them. You will be kneeling on a pad that will lift your body up and down so the more weight you set on the weight stack, the easier it makes the dip. The weight stack works essentially like a counterweight to your body weight.

There are two ways you can do this one. If you are concerned mostly with building massive triceps, you need to keep your body as vertical as possible while performing this exercise. If you want to put more stress on the chest muscles, then lean forward. That's the only change. Because this exercise works the chest and the triceps, it works wonderfully as a transition from your chest routine to your triceps routine if you have a chest and triceps day. Love it. Watch the videos at www.gandmfitness.ca/startrightvideos.

CHINS OR PULL-UPS

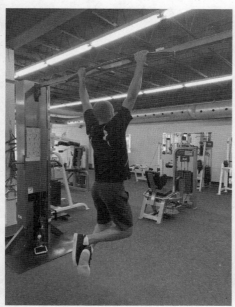 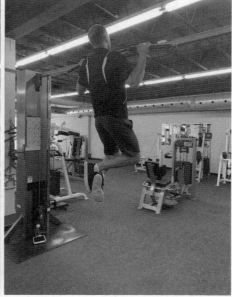

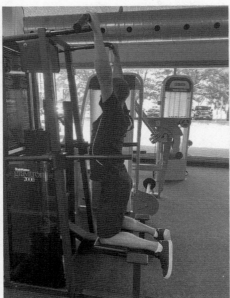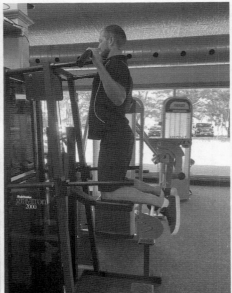

Introduction

This is another great compound movement to help build an impressive back!

Muscles Involved

The primary movers in this one are your latissimus dorsi (lats) and rhomboids—pretty much your whole back musculature—with the help of your biceps as a secondary mover.

Technique

If you choose to do this one, it will obviously be done as part of your back routine, and you will do this one first. If your gym has a Gravitron machine, as ours does, you are in luck because it too has a chin-up bar, so you can use the counterweight to enable you to do the required amount of repetitions, and as you get stronger and are able to do more than the ten to twelve reps, you can lessen the weight to provide you with less counterbalance, thus making the movement more challenging. If your gym does not have a Gravitron, you'll need help with this one in order to get the most benefit. Whether it is just a friend in the gym or a partner, you need that person to hold your feet back behind you while you are doing this movement in order to keep your body vertical to the floor. Without the help of this person, you will inevitably end up curling your body forward which will place more load on the biceps and less on your back. So if you are alone and have no help, just try to do as many as you can, keeping your body as vertical as you can, as long as you can, and add the seated pull-downs to the routine right after you do your pull-ups. The way to increase the load on this one is to use the same belt you used with your dip exercise. So, you have several options with this exercise. Pay attention to your hand positioning. You should know by now where to place your hands if you've been paying attention. Watch the videos at www.gandmfitness.ca/startrightvideos.

PULLOVERS

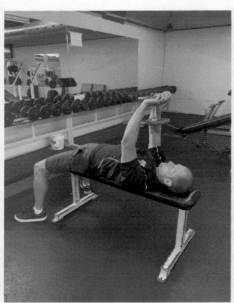 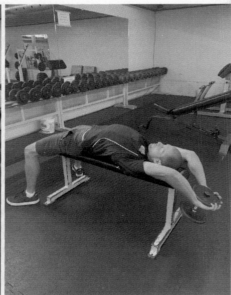

Introduction

This is one of my absolute favourites. This is another great compound exercise, and hardly anyone does this one. I don't recall seeing anyone doing this one in my gym—or any other gym, for that matter—which is unfortunate because it is such a great exercise and works so many upper body muscles.

Muscles Involved

More specifically, this exercise works the traps, the lats, the chest, and the triceps. I love them. I think the reason most don't do this one is that if you don't learn to do this one properly and give it a chance, you won't be comfortable, you'll stop doing them, and thus you won't realize the benefit. You can do this one on chest day or back day; it doesn't matter because it works both very intensely.

Technique

In order to do this one properly, first you need to realize that this is a one-joint movement—the shoulder joint. Your elbow joint will bend slightly as you stretch your arms downward behind your head towards the floor, but it's the shoulder joint that will be mostly involved. So, lying on a flat bench cupping a dumbbell in your hands, the starting position will be above your chest, arms extended straight up, vertical and perpendicular to the floor, with soft elbows. Slowly bring the dumbbell down behind your head towards the floor until you get a great stretch in your lats and chest and triceps, so the bottom position will be when the dumbbell is behind your head and almost touching the floor with elbows just slightly bent and pointing upwards towards the ceiling. You must feel comfortable here in this bottom position. If you are not, it's likely because your arms are extended too far out. Once in this bottom position, lift the dumbbell back up to the starting position above your chest. Remember not to lock out your elbows at the top. Watch the video at www.gandmfitness.ca/startrightvideos.

SQUATS

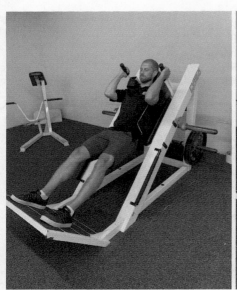
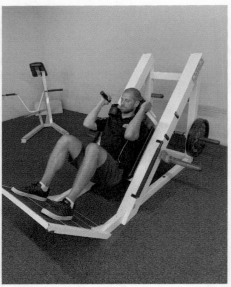
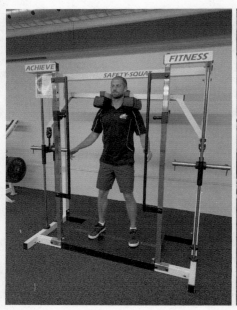
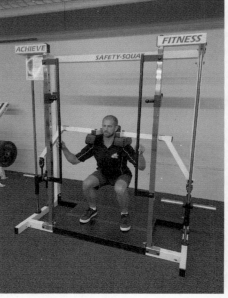

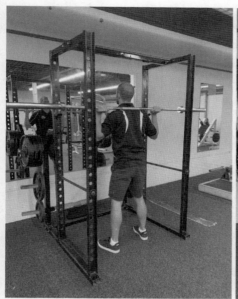 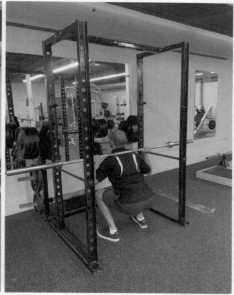

Introduction

I have a lot to say about this one. If you can learn to love this one half as much as I do, and do them consistently and correctly, you'll be doing yourself a great service. This one will create for you a set of very strong legs that will serve you for the rest of your life. As you age, you will inevitably lose strength all over your body. It's a natural part of aging, but if you are strength training, it will be as minimal as possible. The first and most common issue elderly people that don't strength train encounter is loss of strength in their legs. They start having trouble with stairs, getting in and out of their cars, getting up and down off of the ground to do things like gardening and playing with their grandchildren, and so on. Quite a few end up using either a cane or a walker, which in my opinion is completely avoidable. Don't let that person with the cane or walker be you. When I visited my parents' home town in Southern Italy, I didn't see any seniors using canes or walkers. There was no such thing. Can you guess why? This town was situated on the side of a mountain. These people, all of their lives, were either walking uphill or downhill, or usually both, every day, multiple times a day. There were no cars or bikes. They walked everywhere, many times for hours. They developed very strong leg muscles, which, as I mentioned, served them very well, deep into their senior years. It was quite normal to see an eighty-nine-year-old person walking up a steep hill with not much effort at all, and here in North America, our seniors can barely make it up a flight of stairs with the help of a handrail! As I said, it's unfortunate and, in my opinion, unnecessary if you do what is needed to avoid that happening to you before it happens.

Muscles Involved

On that note, on with what is necessary: the squat. First of all, the squat movement involves several muscle groups in order to perform it properly. It is actually one of the only compound exercises that require two or more opposing muscle groups to contract (shorten) at the same time! Your quadriceps in front of your thighs and your hamstring muscles in the back of your thighs and your gluteus maximus all must contract at the same time in order for you to launch yourself out of a full squatting position.

Technique

I don't recommend, if you are just starting out, that you jump right into squats. You've done the leg press now for a few months, at least as one of the basic exercises, so if you've done them properly and to muscle failure as I've described, you should be ready for the next step towards the squat. The next step, as we do at our club, is get you to actually stand up and do an exercise similar to squats; these are done in a machine called the hack squat. This machine gets you to press with your legs similar to the leg press, but now you are on your feet with the resistance on your legs and glutes. It's a bit closer to the actual squat, but not quite a free-weight squat. Next, after a month or two of hack squats, we would progress to the safety squat machine. This machine mimics the actual squat but has rails to hang on to for balance. After a month or two there, we would advance to free-weight squats, as we would consider you as ready as you'll ever be. If your gym has these two machines, use them first. You'll then be better prepared to do the real free-weight squats. If your gym does not have them, well, you'll just have to suck it up and proceed to the free-weight squat very carefully.

Squats take a lot of effort, take a lot out of you, and take some time to perfect the form necessary to do them as intended. Although the movement is quite natural, the problem is that most try too hard and end up turning a simple, natural movement into something complicated and uncomfortable. In addition to the video, here are my written instructions as best as I can give you. Once you've read these instructions and watched the video, you will need to practice the form with only the Olympic bar on your shoulders until you feel comfortable performing the movement and are confident that you are doing it correctly. Then, and only then, should you start adding weight to the bar. If you feel any stress on your low back at all, you are not performing the squat correctly. Keep practicing. Remember, you are pressing the weight up with your legs, not your back. Find a squat rack, preferably a power rack. You will set the bar on the rack hooks so that the bar is just below the height of your neck so that you can get underneath the bar with knees bent and be able to stand up with it and it clears the resting hooks. Make sure you are situated in the center of the bar. If you are not, the bar will not balance properly on your shoulders. Also, the bar should rest on your traps, not your neck, so here's a quick tip for you. Once you are in position under the bar, slide your hands in towards your head as far as possible. This will automatically cause your upper traps to contract and lift to provide you with a bigger and thicker pad, so to speak, for the bar to rest on. You can also use a bar pad around the bar for more comfort. If you are using a power rack, you can set the bottom bars to just below where the bar would end up in your bottom position of the squat so that if something goes wrong, you can rest the bar on the rack bars and bow out. Once you stand up with the bar on your shoulders, it is you and only you that will be controlling the bar, so focus. Step back so that when you squat down, the bar will not hit the rack or hooks in any way. Once you are in position, place your feet at shoulder width apart, toes pointed slightly outwards. This will help you balance. With your chin up and chest out, squat down as if you were taking a picture of a toddler or a flower or a dog or cat sitting on the floor. Again, it's a very natural movement, so don't think about it too much here—just do it. Arch your back, chin up, chest out, and down you go. Once your thighs are parallel to the floor, drive back up with your legs, chin up, chest out, and stand back up. Keep your knees just slightly bent and repeat. Nice and slow going down with control and nice and slow back up. Practice, practice, practice, until you can do them with your eyes closed. You will always do these squats facing a mirror. The mirror is there so that you can check your form and body position at all times while performing your sets, not to check your hair or the hot little number working out behind you. Watch the video at www.gandmfitness.ca/startrightvideos.

LYING TRICEP EXTENSIONS OR "HEAD CAVERS"

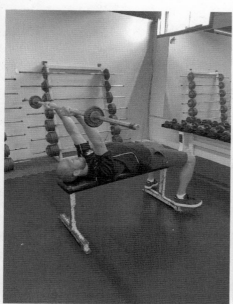 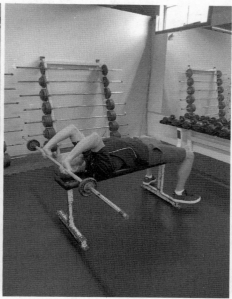

Introduction

This is one of those exercises that are so effective, but only if you are doing it correctly; unfortunately, most don't. I guess it's not a matter of doing it wrong; rather, it's a matter of doing this one in a way in which it will reap the most benefit for you. It's one of those little adjustments that I make to really get the most out of this one that not many are aware of. As I mentioned in an earlier chapter, your body, if you are not paying attention, will do whatever it takes to make an exercise easier to do, and this exercise is a perfect example. First, I'll describe to you how this one is typically done by most everyone, until I see them, and then it's all over. Then, I'll describe how it should be done. When I see a veteran lifter doing it the way everyone typically does it, and I show them how I would prefer them to do it, they are quite happy to discover a more effective way of doing the exercise, but they are very angry because they couldn't lift anywhere near the weight they were using before doing it "my way."

Muscles Involved

This is an isolation exercise that targets only the triceps if done properly. In most cases, doing an exercise properly, with proper form, controlled movement, focus, and using a full range of motion without any loss of load is usually the hardest way to do exercises, not the easiest.

Technique

So, here's how most lifters do this one. You grab a pre-loaded straight bar or e-z curl bar, say twenty-five pounds or so to start. You lie back on a flat bench and press the bar straight off your chest to the straight, locked arm position above your chest. This is the starting position. With your elbows pointing towards your feet, you slowly let your elbows bend and lower the bar with control until just before it bashes into your forehead. Be careful to choose a weight that you can handle, or you are going to find out very quickly why this one is nicknamed "head caver." Stop just before you cave your head in, and then press the weight back up to the straight-arm, vertical, locked position, perpendicular to the floor. Repeat to muscle failure and be very, very careful, especially letting the weight down towards your head, especially those last few, more challenging repetitions.

Here are the issues with this common way of doing this exercise in this manner. First of all (and you should have picked this one up right away) is that at the top of the movement, you are in a locked-arm position, which takes the load off of the triceps between each repetition. We know by now that this is not ideal. Second, when you bring the bar down from the vertical position, the bottom of the movement will be with the bar just an inch or so from your forehead. Again, this is very dangerous. My way of doing this exercise eliminates both issues and makes this exercise by leaps and bounds more effective and much more challenging.

Here it is. Start the same way as was just described, with your arms straight up and vertical, holding the bar in the locked-arm position. This starting position will now change. First, place your thumb underneath the bar alongside the other fingers so as to create a pad with the palm of your hands that the bar will rest on. Next, with your arms still straight, tilt your arms back so that the bar is now above your forehead. This positioning will automatically release the lock on the elbows because of the angle of your arms. You will feel that the weight is trying to bend your elbows now, rather than sitting directly above your locked elbow. With your elbows facing your feet again, slowly lower the bar down to the bottom position without changing the angle of your upper arm. It remains still, and tilted back. You will notice now that because your starting position was further back above your forehead instead of above your chest that the bottom position is now behind your head rather than above your forehead. Danger averted. Press the weight back to the start position, which is now with your straight-arm position angled back. Do not return to the vertical, elbows-locked position above your chest. Once you try it this way, you will feel how challenging this one really is and should be. Big, big difference with just a few minor adjustments. Veterans take note! Watch the video at www.gandmfitness.ca/startrightvideos.

INCLINE DUMBBELL PRESS

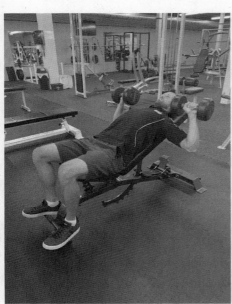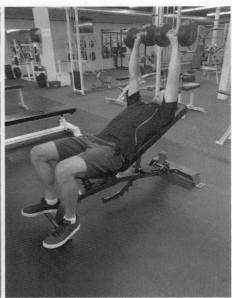

Introduction

This is definitely another one of my favourites, and I still do this one as the first exercise in every chest workout. Before I describe the proper form, you'll need to understand why this particular version of the chest press is, in my opinion, the best chest exercise that you can do. If you think about it, up until now, the chest exercises, whether it be the vertical chest press, the flat dumbbell press, or the flat bench press, all place your body in the same position in relation to your pressing movement. That is to say that you are pressing straight off of your chest, vertical to your body. Remember this: in most cases, the pectoral muscle has most of its mass in the lower half of the pectoral muscles.

Muscles Involved

As such, in this particular exercise, your body will be inclined (your head higher than your hips) which involves more of the upper portion of the chest muscles with some help from the front deltoid (shoulder) muscles. So, in order to place more stress on the upper half of the chest muscle, you need to do the pressing movement with your body angled at an incline, thus the name incline dumbbell press.

Technique

You will find, at any gym that offers a free-weight area, an adjustable incline bench. This bench will allow you to set the backrest at pretty much any angle you want. Set it at about thirty-five degrees, which, if you look at it from the side, is less than halfway between flat and straight upright. When you are lying in this position with dumbbells in hand, you will still be pressing straight up off the floor. The tendency here is to naturally press straight up off of your chest, but that's not correct, or comfortable, for that matter. So, although your instinct is to just press straight off of your chest, you are going to focus, and press straight up towards the ceiling. This angle will provide most of the stress on the upper portion of the chest muscles, thereby developing more mass there, and will result in a much nicer development of the chest all around. So, I would start with this one, and then choose a flat version of the chest press as your second exercise. Add something like the pec deck or chest flys as a third exercise, and your chest routine is over. If you are doing triceps after chest, this would be a perfect time to do the dips described earlier as a transition from chest to triceps.

In my professional opinion, you should consider using dumbbells instead of the bar whenever you can. The reason is that using a bar all of the time for your presses, whether it be for chest presses or shoulder presses, will place a ton of unnecessary stress across your upper body, and more specifically your shoulders. In time, you will experience shoulder issues because of it. When you use dumbbells, it allows your shoulders to work independently of each other, thereby eliminating that stress across the front of your upper body. Dumbbells rule, in my book. Watch the video at www.gandmfitness.ca/startrightvideos.

SHOULDER SHRUGS

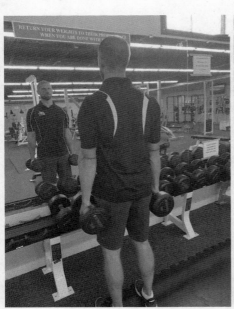
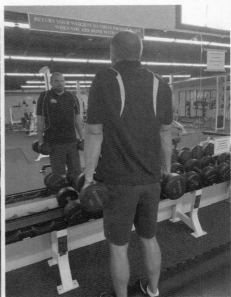

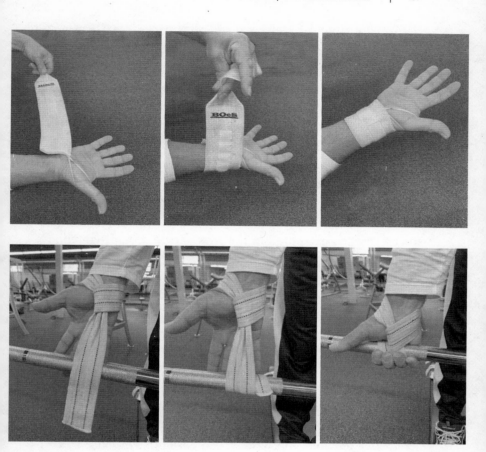

Introduction

This is a very simple movement, but nevertheless essential. It should be a part of every shoulder or back routine.

Muscles Involved

The shoulder shrug isolates the trapezius muscle, which, if you look at yourself in the mirror, is the bump on each side of your neck that runs from the bottom of your neck to the top of your shoulders. What most don't realize is that this muscle also runs more than halfway down your back. It starts as a wide muscle at the top of your back and tapers down to a very narrow area about three-quarters of the way down your back, essentially forming a triangle shape. Because this movement is quite easy to perform, you will find that you will be able to use quite a bit of weight with this one, so this would be a great opportunity to try out some wrist straps. I'll throw in a video on how to use wrist straps because a lot of times I see people using them backwards. The straps should help you hang on to the dumbbells for as long as you need to unless you are using them incorrectly. As your grip starts to falter and your fingers start to extend a bit, the wrist straps should tighten, not loosen.

Technique

You will be standing with good posture, arms hanging naturally at your sides, with dumbbells in hand, and you will simply raise or shrug your shoulders as high as you can and then slowly lower your shoulders back to the start position. **Do not rotate your shoulders.** Straight up and down is the correct and safest way to do this exercise, and don't let anyone tell you otherwise. When doing this exercise in a standing, upright body position, it will primarily isolate the upper portion of the traps, which is the part you see when you look in the mirror. The mid and lower portion of this muscle will get its workout with the rowing movements that you will do on back day. You can also isolate the mid and lower portions of this muscle by sitting on the end of a flat bench, and rather than sitting up straight and perpendicular to the floor, you will lean forward with your upper body, arms still hanging naturally, while still maintaining good posture. This position will move the load down your back. One last suggestion is to do this one right in front of the dumbbell rack so you can grab the set of dumbbells that you want to use, step back, sitting or standing, do your set, and then place the dumbbells right back on the rack where you got them from. No need to walk off somewhere with the dumbbells to a place where you can do this exercise off of a bench, or worse yet, off of the floor; that's just silly. Watch the videos at www.gandmfitness.ca/startrightvideos.

CLOSE GRIP BENCH PRESS

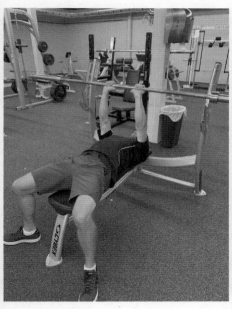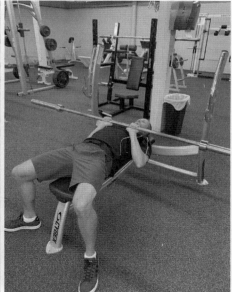

Introduction and Muscles Involved

This is a great tricep builder. The only difference between this exercise and the flat bench press described earlier is the placement of your grip on the bar. The closer your hands are together, the more work your triceps will have to do to press the weight off of your chest. Remember, it's the exercises that you can use a lot of weight with that are the best ones to build muscle mass, so this one is right up there. Keep in mind that although we are going to use a close grip, too close is no good either.

Technique

So as you lie on the flat bench, place your hands on the bar with your thumbs along the bottom of the bar as spacers. Slide your hands together until your thumbs are about four or five inches apart. That's close enough. The problem with placing your hands too close together is that it will be almost impossible to balance the bar, and your wrists will pay the price. By placing your grip the way I described, you will lift the bar off the forks with care to control the balance of the bar, and lower the bar keeping your arms at your sides. This will cause your elbows to completely collapse, thus making the triceps the prime movers responsible for pressing the bar back up to the top, "soft elbow" position. Watch the video at www.gandmfitness.ca/startrightvideos.

There are more really good advanced exercises, but the ones I've just described are among my favourites and should be included in your workout routine if you are interested in building muscle mass as efficiently and effectively as possible.

NOT A PLAYGROUND

Assuming that you are reading this chapter for exactly that reason, I'm going to share with you now one of the realities of being an advanced weightlifter and thus using heavy weights most days of the week. It can be very dangerous if you are not paying attention! I'll say that again. It can be very dangerous if you are not paying attention. It's the same as the butcher example I gave earlier in the book when I was writing about focus. It's the same as a machine operator not paying attention. Some of the memories that I have stuck in my head of my days working in the machine shop for years as a machinist were not very nice ones. A few of the machinists I met that became my very good friends were missing fingers! And also, once in a while, the ambulance would show up because someone who was not paying attention would shear off their fingers on the shearing machine.

Once, and this happened to me personally, I was drilling a part on the gang drill, and I was using a long extension drill bit because I had a long hole to drill in this particular part. That extension drill bit rotating at over one-thousand RPMs (revolutions per minute) hit the edge of the jig and broke. Guess where the broken piece of drill bit ended up? It flew across the shop and went right through my buddy's chin into his mouth. True story.

The gym is no different. Here are some of the things that I have witnessed first-hand in my own gym over the years, believe it or not.

Remember the flat dumbbell presses I described earlier in the book? Well, one day, a member decided to choose a weight that he obviously couldn't handle, so as he reached the top of the movement with his arms extended, his one elbow joint gave out, and that dumbbell came crashing down right on his face. The dumbbell survived, and I'm not referring to the weight.

Another time, I was working out, minding my own business, when I spotted a guy at the squat rack loading what seemed to me to be way too much weight for a guy of his stature, so I watched carefully as I had a sneaking suspicion that this wasn't going to end well—and it didn't. He proceeded to get under the bar and stand up with it on his shoulders, and he stepped back ready to do his set. I noticed right away that his legs were already shaking, and he hadn't even done one repetition yet! He was just standing there, weight on his shoulders. I thought he was just going to give it up and place the bar back on the rack, but he didn't. What happened next is hard to believe, even for me. He squatted down with the weight on his shoulders and could not get back up. He had no spotter to help him. His back was bending forward under the weight, and I guess the only way he thought he could get out of that situation was to drop the load on the floor, so he bent forward even more, head down, and let the bar roll off of him onto the floor, nearly ripping his head off on the way down. I could not believe what I had just seen.

Another time a member doing tricep pushdowns on a cable machine got too close to the cable with his face, and as he let the weight stack down at the end of his set and the handle went up past his face, the S-hook that attached the handle to the cable caught the one side of his nose and ripped right through it. What a bloody mess that was.

Another time, a member not paying attention was loading the Olympic bar on the squat rack, preparing to do his next set of squats. Because he was not paying attention, he loaded one extra plate on one side of the bar, making it unbalanced. He got under the bar and stood up straight to lift the weight off of the rack, and you can imagine what happened next. Because he wasn't using collars to hold the weights in place on the bar, and the one side had forty-five more pounds on it than the other side, the lighter side went up, causing all of the weights on the heavy side to slide off, and then all of the weights on the lighter side, along with the bar, flipped and fell onto the floor. If that last bunch of weights and the bar had hit anyone as it flipped off the squat rack, it could have seriously hurt or even killed someone.

Another time, same squat rack, different member—not paying attention again—was stripping the weights off of the bar to put them away back on the storage pins of the rack. The problem was that he was taking all of the weight plates off of the one side without taking any off of the other side. Once he slid the last plate off of the bar on the one side, you guessed it, the bar went flying up and just missed taking his head off as all of the weights and the bar went crashing down on the other side of the rack. That was a close call. That's a lesson for you readers. Now you know: you take one plate off of one side and then one off of the other, and repeat until all weights are off the bar.

I've dealt with people falling off the back extension machine onto the floor, dislocated shoulders, and crushed toes from dropping a dumbbell on them. I've dealt with young high school girls fainting (several times) because they hadn't eaten all day and did an exercise routine without any energy at all. I got so good at spotting the potential fainting victim that I actually caught the last one in my arms before she hit the floor. I've dealt with anorexia, steroid rage, unconsciousness, and even a death.

My point here is this: The weight room is not a playground. It is a serious place to lift weights and is no place for screwing around. Be careful, be alert, and most of all, pay attention to what you are doing, not what others are doing.

DON'T LET YOUR PARTNER GET STUCK

Sooner or later you are going to end up with a partner, and sometimes not by choice—but becoming one's partner is much more than taking on the role of a cheerleader. Of course, a good partner will be there for you to give you positive reinforcement, encouragement, and sometimes a much-needed attitude adjustment. But be forewarned that there is one thing that you need to be aware of that is of utmost importance, and that is the ability to be a good spotter. If you have a partner that really knows how to spot properly, you definitely have an advantage. Your spotter will give you more confidence by you knowing someone is there to help you out if you need it. They will also be there to help you squeeze out a few more repetitions that you would not be able to do safely without them there—which in turn allows you to perform more negatives, right? The worst thing is having a partner spot you that has no knowledge or experience in doing that. If that is the case, don't ask for a spot. Just do what you are able to do on your own. I've seen first-hand what can happen when someone randomly asks another member to spot them, only to find out in the middle of their last repetition that the help that they are expecting is not coming. Big trouble. So, keeping in mind what you learned about being stronger on the negative than on the positive contraction (see chapter 13), you should realize that the help your partner will likely need is only on the positive phase of their lift, so be ready! There is nothing worse than a spotter that is not helping right away when it is required, before the movement stops and the partner gets stuck. You have to anticipate that by paying attention and being ready. Don't let them get stuck. Keep the positive moving, and let them do the negative. That's how it should work.

Spotting a squatter is a whole different ball game. When you are spotting someone that is doing a pressing movement or a curl or a pull-down, things like that, it's pretty easy. You spot them by actually touching the bar or the weight stack, and help as needed. But when you are spotting a person squatting, it gets very close and personal. The only way to spot a squatter properly, in my opinion, whether they like it or not, is to squat up and down with them, directly behind them without touching them, with your arms wrapped around their waist and your hands on their chest. The reason you have to do it this way is that when a squatter runs into trouble driving that weight up, if their legs can't do it, what will happen is their hips will start to raise but their backs won't go up. This is where you need to help raise their upper body and the bar at the same time, and the only way to do that is to have your arms around them and your hands on their chest—like it or not. Here are some pictures and a video that better illustrate what I've just explained. Go to www.gandmfitness.ca/startrightvideos.

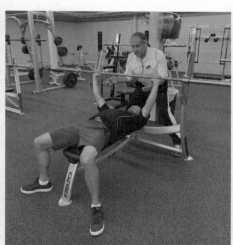
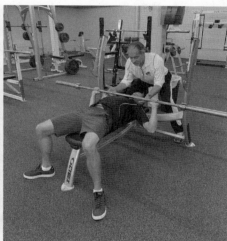
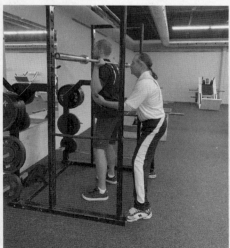
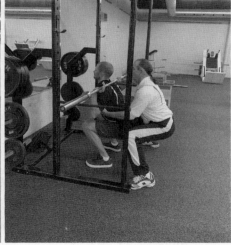

USELESS AND INFERIOR EXERCISES

Lastly, and in closing this chapter on heavy weightlifting, there are several exercises that I see a lot of lifters doing that I consider a waste of time and effort. Sometimes it's because it's just not an effective exercise if you are lifting to gain muscle mass, and sometimes it's just such an inferior exercise to the other exercises they just finished doing that it is rendered useless. Keep in mind that I am addressing those who are interested in building muscle mass, so things like doing lunges after heavy squats is ridiculous, not to mention that you should hardly be able to stand up, let alone do lunges after a great squat routine. So, here we go.

Decline Chest Press

If I got rid of the decline bench press we have at our gym, I would be hung out to dry. The reason is that the members who use it constantly don't realize what a useless exercise it really is. As I mentioned prior, the incline chest press is king in my book, flat presses a close second, but the decline...... useless. Because the angle of your body is declined, (your head lower than your hips), in this position your pectoral muscles are not doing much of anything. If anything, it's the extreme bottom portion of the chest muscles that will be working, the ones that really don't need specific attention because they will develop just as well doing flat presses. The prime movers in this exercise are really your triceps.

Kickbacks

If your intent is to build muscle mass, then the exercises that you choose to include in your workout routines should only be the ones that you can lift a lot of weight with. Kickbacks is not one of them; thus, I deem them useless in a mass-building routine. For those of you who don't know what kickbacks are, it's the exercise where you are standing bent over, upper arm held parallel to the floor, elbow at ninety degrees, and you are holding on to a dumbbell in your hand. The other arm is supporting you somehow by holding on to the side of a machine or resting on top of the dumbbell rack. You try to extend your bent arm without moving your upper arm position until it is straight and then return to the ninety-degree position. How much weight can one possibly use for this exercise? Five pounds, eight pounds, maybe ten pounds? Now, ask yourself how much weight you can use doing dips, head cavers, and tricep pushdowns. A lot more, rendering this exercise useless for muscle gains. Don't waste your time.

Standing Straight Arm Side Lateral Raises

This is a great shoulder exercise for beginners, and it's how we start most of our new clients. It does its job at the start. Once you are at a level where you are looking for the advanced exercises to help build that mass you are looking for in your shoulders, drop this one. This is one of those exercises that are effective to a point, but then, you just aren't able to use a lot of weight, enough to initiate that muscle growth process of breaking down the muscle and resting, recuperating, and adapting. The reason you can't increase the weight resistance much with this exercise is that with a straight arm, the shoulder muscles—more specifically, the medial deltoid, which is the prime mover—is very short in relation to where the weight-bearing dumbbell is located: way down at the end of your arm, so as such is at a huge disadvantage, thus limiting the amount of load that you can lift with proper form. To illustrate better, picture yourself trying to lift a shovel full of snow or dirt with both your hands at the top of the shovel barely six inches apart. That would be very difficult, but if you move your one hand down the shaft of the shovel, now you have moved the lifting point down closer to the load, making the lift much easier. Now, having said that, if your gym has a seated side lateral raise machine like ours does, wow, use it. In my opinion, that particular machine is the best thing you can use to build strong and big medial deltoid muscles without having to press anything over your head. The pads that you are pushing against on this machine are located on the forearm and elbow joint, much closer to where the deltoid attaches to the upper arm, and you are sitting up vertical. I love it. Go to www.gandmfitness.ca/startrightvideos to watch the video.

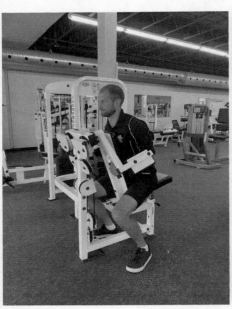
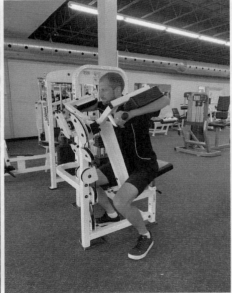

Abductor/Adductor Exercises

Leave this one for your yoga class. It is such an inferior exercise compared to a squat or a leg press that it's nothing but a waste of time and effort if you are training for muscle mass in your legs. Period.

Now, don't get me wrong. All exercises are beneficial in one way or another. You just have to always keep in mind what it is that you are training for, so you need to recognize the exercises that will get you where you want to be in the most effective and efficient way possible.

NOTES

BONUS CHAPTER 2:
A Few Words about Performance-Enhancing Supplements and Drugs

This chapter is written specifically to address the temptation that will inevitably rear its ugly head in most gyms if you are one of those eager adolescents that have one thing in mind, increasing muscle size. The temptation to build a muscular physique as quickly as possible, no matter what the consequences, is common, and some are actually willing to risk their good health to build big muscles fast.

Sooner or later, it will become obvious to you that certain individuals in the gym will get very big and strong far more quickly than anyone else. Are they working harder? Are they just natural athletes? Do they just have good genes? Do they know some secret exercises that I'm not aware of? The answer to all of those questions is "no."

The reality of it is that most humans want everything to happen now, as soon as possible, and unfortunately with as little effort as possible. The other reality is that in bodybuilding and strength training, it's easier than you think, but comes with great risk to your good health.

Enter the performance-enhancing drugs. Believe it or not, they are everywhere and easily accessible. Believe me when I tell you that there are members in every single gym that are either using them, selling them, or typically both.

I can't with a clear conscience write a book about strength training and joining a gym without addressing this issue, especially for the young in body and young at heart. If there is anyone reading this book that is taking up strength training and joining a gym that is at all skeptical about whether or not one can build good, solid muscle without the use of dangerous, illegal, performance-enhancing drugs, have a look at the picture at the end of the book. That's me—a lifetime natural, amateur body builder.

I've spent most of my adult life weightlifting, strength training, and bodybuilding. Have I ever been tempted to use drugs to help me? Of course I have, many, many times. Did I give in? No way. If I had, that would have made me the biggest hypocrite in my gym. I consider myself a lifetime, natural amateur bodybuilder, and damn proud of it. The muscle you will build as a natural bodybuilder is just that—natural. And as such, it will stay with you long into your senior years, not to mention serve you well in regard to your general health. The opposite is true by building muscle the other way. The muscles you are building are not natural, will not stay with you unless you continue to use those drugs indefinitely, and are a definite and proven risk to your good health.

If you recall, in chapter 11 I touched on the hormone cortisol and its responsibility for protecting the human body from growing too much muscle. Well, guess which hormone is suppressed by those performance-enhancing drugs? Cortisol. That's one reason for the unnatural growth of muscle experienced by those who use them. So, if you see someone that has unnaturally big muscles and are wondering if they use performance-enhancing drugs, they do. End of story.

Ask yourself this question: Are you willing to risk your good health at such an early age, just to build muscle more quickly than most, when you know that you can eventually do it naturally, like I did, and not risk a possible life-threatening disease? I should think not. So, don't listen to Nike and "just do it"; listen to me and "just don't."

I've spoken to doctors about this, and several of them, and I've witnessed first-hand the issues that those choosing to use those drugs have had to endure, and I assure you that those are issues you do not want to experience at a young age, or any age, for that matter. I've even known a few that have passed away as a direct result of abusing themselves by using these drugs. Don't do it.

Furthermore—and this is important!—if you think that what these members are buying off of the street is pure and safe, think again. Like most black market drugs, they are mostly diluted, and the majority of them are fake. Trust me when I tell you that you can't afford the real stuff anyway, so forget all about it and train as I'm teaching you here, with a clear conscience and your good health.

As far as supplements are concerned, here's my take.

I've only found one natural supplement over all these years that actually makes your muscles physically bigger (because this supplement forces your muscle cells to hold more water), and it actually makes you stronger by helping your muscle fibres to contract more efficiently. It's natural and it's safe. It's called Creatine. If you choose to supplement with this product for longer than three months, you should have your Creatinine level checked, as the by-product of Creatine is Creatinine and may build up on you. I have good, reliable studies that show no negative side effects from the use of Creatine.

I would also recommend a high-quality multivitamin and a high-quality protein powder.

It seems to me that all of the other supplements that are sold at gyms are generally stimulants, created to give you a boost of energy so that you can get a better, more energetic workout. If that is something you think you need, then do some research and choose carefully. (And don't forget to consider buying it from your gym first!)

NOTES

BONUS CHAPTER 3:
Putting Together Your Own Advanced Workouts

If you are reading this chapter, you've got the bug. You are now considered to be a "gym rat." You've gone through all of the basic stuff, taken my advice, and prepared yourself properly. Now, you are ready to train like a pro.

The information you are about to read is certainly available from a good trainer, but I understand that there are a lot of reasons why people will not or cannot hire a personal trainer, so hopefully, this chapter will be enough to guide you in constructing your own more advanced routines yourself.

This information should also bring to light all that is involved from a personal trainer's perspective concerning designing an appropriate training program for their clients. There's a lot more to it than most realize, so I'm happy to offer this information to bring that required effort to the forefront.

Prior to actually giving you the suggested split routines that you can try, I'm going to cover all of the important issues when faced with the challenge of designing a proper, effective, and efficient training program. That way, you will be able to better understand why the split routines are designed the way they are.

WORKOUT DURATION

Make certain that your entire weight training portion of the workout takes no longer than one hour. Preferably forty-five minutes. You should be able to recall why, as I explained this in chapter 11. Remember the hormone cortisol, and the limiting and protective effects of the hormone cortisol? If you don't, go back and reread bonus chapter 2.

REST DAYS

Remember how important proper rest and recuperation is to your results? My suggestion and rule of thumb is that if you've weight trained for three consecutive days, the fourth day should be a complete rest day from any weightlifting. If you then resume and weight train for another three consecutive days, then the fourth day and fifth day should be rest days. I know what you are thinking and stop thinking that way. You need those rest days. If you are training as hard as you should be, you need them!

BALANCE

Keep in mind the issue of balance. We discussed the importance of keeping a balanced workout routine in chapter 10 and bonus chapter 1. If you fall into the same trap as a lot of lifters and do not address this concern when constructing your workouts, be prepared for shoulder pain, knee pain, back pain, elbow pain, hip pain, and more.

ORDER OF WORKOUTS

Don't let the workout you are doing today negatively affect the workout you will do tomorrow. Let me explain. As I mentioned in chapter 10, unless you are doing an isolation exercise, all other exercises, the compound exercises, the most important ones, have a prime mover and a secondary mover. Let's take the chest press as an example. The prime movers in this instance are the pectoral (chest) muscles, and the secondary movers are the triceps and front deltoids. You would not want to train your triceps or front deltoids the day before your chest workout. If you do, your triceps and front deltoids will not be able to help complete the lift as well as if you had well-rested, recuperated triceps and delts to contribute to the all-important compound exercise like the bench press. Another great example would be to not train your biceps the day before your back workout. Same reason. You need fresh, well-rested, and recuperated biceps to help with the all-important back exercises. There is a principle called pre-exhausting that basically says that if you pre-exhaust or tire the secondary movers, this will force the primary movers to work alone and it's harder to lift the weight, thus resulting in a better result. I strongly disagree. At the end of the day, the benefit comes from lifting as heavy as you can properly, and pre-exhausting a secondary mover, in my opinion, is counterproductive.

ORDER OF EXERCISES

If you understood what I tried to explain in the previous paragraph, you will understand this one. It's the same issue. Why would you do a tricep routine and then do your chest routine right after in the same workout? You would do it the other way around, obviously. If you don't, well, you may be the next dumbbell to have a dumbbell crash into your face because your triceps gave out! Don't be that person. So, the large prime movers get trained first, then the secondary next—never the other way around.

Another point regarding order of exercises that I can make here is to prioritize the compound movements. So, for example, if you are training your legs, you would place your squats or leg press as the first exercise, and then if you so choose can add things like hamstring curls, leg extensions, calf raises, and so on. Same thing applies to any large muscle groups that are best trained with compound exercises like the chest presses, shoulder presses, chins, and so on. Do the compound exercise first, and then the isolation exercises like front deltoid raises, rear deltoid flys, pectoral flys, and so on.

HEAVY LIFTING

By now, you should be ready for the real heavy stuff, but let me remind you again: heavy weights can be dangerous, so pay attention! At this stage in your training, and keeping in mind why you are doing this, you need to choose exercises that you can use heavy weights with. So, forget about the kick-backs, the wrist curls, the standing straight-arm lateral raises, the one-arm pushdowns for triceps, the abductor/adductor exercises, the knee raises, the hip extensions for gluteals, the oblique exercises, the straight-arm pushdowns, and do consider including exercises like the incline dumbbell presses, dumbbell shoulder presses, squats, leg presses, chins, rows, shrugs, standing calf raises, dips, and so on.

UNSUPPORTED FORWARD FLEXION

Allow me a brief word about deadlifts. If you've noticed, this is the first time in this entire book that I've mentioned deadlifts. There's a reason, and a good one. Deadlifts are very high-risk and very dangerous to your low back. What I've experienced and witnessed over the past thirty-five years is that most, if not all, of the people that have included deadlifts in their workouts have ended up injuring themselves sooner or later—and I'm talking about veteran lifters, not beginners. Again, in my opinion, the risk of injury is not worth the effort or the results. There are many safer ways to get the same results. Furthermore, the fitness industry has taught us that these types of exercises are considered "contraindicated," which basically means, "Dangerous—don't do them, and if you do choose to do them, be very, very careful." They are considered dangerous because they demonstrate perfectly what unsupported forward flexion is. Any time you bend forward to pick something up without leaning on something for support is considered unsupported forward flexion. It is very dangerous to your low back. The simple movement of just bending over without support causes tremendous stress on your low back, without even picking anything up! Can you imagine the stress on the low back if you did that with hundreds of pounds of weight on an Olympic bar? It's unnecessary, and I'll go as far as to say foolish, to risk your back health in that manner. Furthermore, once you've injured your low back by doing something like that, it'll haunt you for the rest of your days. Consider yourself warned.

SPLIT ROUTINES AND HOW TO CREATE THEM

Here are some sample split routines, most of which I've done myself for years. I'll place them in a progressive order so that when you are ready, you can start with the first one, and every three months or so progress to the next.

Two-Day Split Routine

Day One: Chest, back and biceps. Day Two: Legs, shoulders and triceps. I did this split for a long, long time because I loved it. I loved it so much because I was very young, and I didn't want to work out at the gym on the weekends, especially in the summer, so Day One was Mondays, Day Two was on Tuesday, Wednesday was off, Thursday was Day One again, Friday was Day Two again and I took the weekend off. I loved it. I spent most of those weekends on the beach. Keep in mind that with this first split, you can only do two exercises per body part, or the workout will take too long, so pick the good ones. Add calves and abs to whichever day you want. As you progress to more splits, you can add more exercises per body part because you will be working less body parts. Get it? Good. Here's a typical two-day split routine. Day One: Incline dumbbell press and pec deck for chest, then pull-downs and rows for back, then standing barbell curls and preacher curls for biceps, then crunches for abs. Done. Day Two: Squats or leg press for legs, then seated dumbbell press and rear delt flys for shoulders, then head cavers and pushdowns for triceps, then standing calf raises for calves. Done.

Three-Day Split Routine

I loved this one just as much as the first one because here, you are only working two body parts per workout, so you can do three exercises per body part, which will prove to make a noticeable change in results to your physique. Remember now, the harder you work, the more rest you will need. So having said that, once you progress to this and the following splits, there is no such thing as "days of the week" any longer. That is out the window. It's just Day One, Day Two, Day Three, and so on, regardless of what day of the week it is. Every week will be different. It's also going to start to seem like you are not working those muscle groups often enough, but you are, so trust me. A typical three-day split routine would be something like this: Day One would be chest and triceps, then Day Two would be back and biceps, then Day Three would be legs and shoulders, then two days off, so that would mean that if you started this split on a Monday, you would be starting over again on Saturday with Day One, so you can see how the days of the week are no longer relevant. The other nice thing about being at this stage is that if you miss a workout day for whatever reason, so what? Consider it more rest and recuperation. Here's what the actual workouts may consist of. Day One: Incline dumbbell press, then flat bench press, then dips for chest, and then close grip presses, head cavers and pushdowns for triceps. Day Two: Chins or pull-downs, seated vertical row, and then one-arm rows for back, then standing barbell curls, preacher curls, and incline dumbbell curls for biceps. Day Three: Squats or leg press, then hamstring curls and standing calf raises for legs, seated dumbbell presses, rear delt flys and heavy shrugs for shoulders, and then crunches for abs. Done. The first thing you will notice is that these workouts are a lot of work. At this stage, you should be taking two days off after every three days. Write down on a calendar what workout day it is because you are going to lose track if you don't, trust me. I did more than once. Also, because of the amount of work involved now at this stage, you may feel that you need more than two days off, and if you feel you do, take an extra day. You know I won't object. On those rest days, all you need to think about is how your body is recuperating and growing, so rest and eat, rest and eat.

Four-Day Split Routine

The only difference between this split and the three-day split routine is that I've created a separate day for legs. Leg day! It's not Day One, Day Two, or Day Three, it's **leg day**!!! Hurray! So, because you have removed the leg portion of your Day Three, you can add another shoulder exercise like upright rows or front raises to your shoulder routine. Be careful with the upright rows, as they are considered another contraindicated exercise. There is a risk of what's called "impingement" of the rotator cuff muscles where the small rotator muscles get pinched under the clavicle bone, but if you have heeded my advice and you have good balance in your shoulder musculature, you should be fine. Have fun!

NOTES

BONUS CHAPTER 4:
Sample Split Routines

Here are some sample split routines that we commonly pre-
scribe at our club for our clients. It will be up to you, now
armed with all of the information you have been given
throughout this book, to choose which type of presses you
would like to use, which type of curls, and so on. Remember
to balance, remember to rest adequately, and work hard. Good
luck, and thank you for purchasing this book. I sincerely hope
that it helps you and thousands of others.

Yours truly,
Gino A. Spada

Two-Day Split Routine (upper body; lower body)

Day One: Upper body. Chest press, dips, shoulder press, vertical row, pull-downs, bicep curls, and tricep extensions.

Day Two: Lower body. Leg press, hamstring curls, standing
calf raises, back extensions, abdominal crunches.

Two-Day Split Routine (pushing; pulling)

Day One: Pushing. Chest press, shoulder press, dips, leg press,
standing calf raises.

Day Two: Pulling. Vertical row, pull-downs, bicep curls, back extensions, abdominal crunches.

Two-Day Split Routine (chest, back, and biceps; legs, shoulders, triceps, and abdominals)

Day One: Chest press, pec deck, vertical row, pull-downs, standing bicep curls, preacher curls, back extensions.

Day Two: Leg press, shoulder press, rear delt flys, head cavers, push-downs, calf raises, abdominal crunches.

Three Day Split Routine (chest, triceps, and abdominals; back and biceps; legs and shoulders)

Day One: Incline chest press, peck deck, dips, head cavers, push downs, abdominal crunches.

Day Two: Low row, pull-downs, one arm row, back extensions, standing barbell curls, preacher curls.

Day Three: Squats, standing calf raises, shoulder press, rear delt flys, shrugs.

Four-Day Split Routine (chest, triceps, and abdominals; back and biceps; shoulders; legs)

Day One and Day Two: Same as above.

Day Three: Shoulders. Shoulder press, front raises, side lateral machine, rear delt flys, shrugs, and abdominals.

Day Four: Legs. Squats, standing calf raises, seated calf raises, back extensions.

NOTES

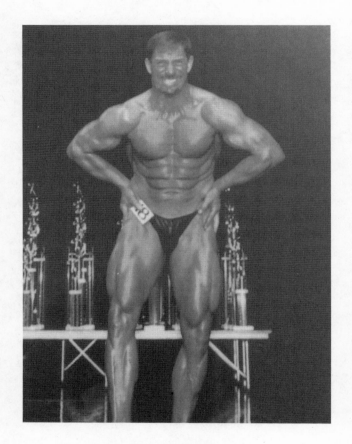

Picture of me.

ABOUT THE AUTHOR

Gino A. Spada was born in May 1960 and raised in Port Colborne, Ontario, Canada. He opened G&M Fitness Health Club in Port Colborne in May 1986. In that year, Gino became a member of the Ontario Fitness Council; was certified in First Aid and CPR; and graduated from the Ontario Fitness Leadership Program (OFLP-YMCA) and the ICS Fitness and Nutrition course.

Gino has coached local ice hockey (house league and travel) from Tyke through to Midget (ages 5 through 17) and is certified as a Level II (Junior Level) Hockey Trainer. His additional certifications include as a Registered Fitness Appraiser by the Canadian Association of Sport Sciences (1987); as a Personal Trainer by the American Council on Exercise (ACE), San Diego, California (1991); and as a Weight Trainer by the International Weight Trainers Association, Ohio (1997). He was also certified by the Health Sciences Academy as a Nutritional Therapist in 2015.

Gino became a competitive amateur natural bodybuilder in 1998 at the age of 38, competing in Buffalo, New York (twice); Rochester, New York; Toronto, Ontario; Hamilton, Ontario; Stratford, Ontario (three times); and Cobourg, Ontario. He has also been a strongman competitor (you haven't lived until you've lifted the back end of a car off the ground—ouch!).

Gino has personally trained hockey players, baseball players, football players, basketball players, soccer players, golfers, swimmers, runners, cyclists, dancers, figure skaters, bodybuilders, power lifters, and many others. He has trained many persons with physical disabilities, including but not limited to those with blindness and paralysis; amputees; victims of motor vehicle accidents; victims of stroke and heart attack; some with chronic fatigue syndrome, fibromyalgia, scoliosis, high blood pressure, diabetes, and arthritis; frail and elderly people; and more.

Gino is recognized as an expert in functional strength training. He is the author of *Eat Smart, Eat Often, Eat Small* ("The S.O.S. Book") (self-published, 2012), a weight management book. He is presently enlisted in the Health Sciences Academy's Harvard-level course Nutrition for Cancer Prevention and Longevity.

Gino has pursued continuing professional education in the following courses: Strength Training and Muscular Endurance (Brock University, St. Catharines, Ontario); Biomechanics of the Upper Body/Biomechanics of the Lower Body (the Nike Network); Personal Training for Seniors (American Senior Fitness Association); Program Design and Exercise Analysis (International Association of Fitness Professionals); Alternative and Complimentary Nutrition Therapy; and Weight Training Injury Symposiums. He has attended every annual Can Fit Pro Conference in Canada since its inception and prior IDEA Conferences. Gino is the original Program Designer for the Ontario Rehabilitation Institute (ORI) in Port Colborne, specializing in post-motor-vehicle-accident rehabilitation.

AWARDS AND ACCOMPLISHMENTS

G&M Fitness was awarded Business of the Quarter in 2006 by the Port Colborne Wainfleet Chamber of Commerce and nominated for Business of the Year in 2006.

Gino was nominated for Citizen of the Year in 2009 and held the position of 3rd Vice President of the Port Colborne Wainfleet Chamber of Commerce in 2008 and 2009.

He was Chairman of the Port Colborne Gateway Association for five years running; served on the Port Colborne Canal Days Committee; and served on the Port Colborne Main Street Revitalization Steering Committee.

Gino is an active real estate investor with nearly a dozen income properties in his portfolio. Besides the health club, he and his family own and operate three retail stores and an online store. Gino is currently retired, but still investing, consulting, training, and overseeing the family businesses and investments.

TRAINER FOR HIRE

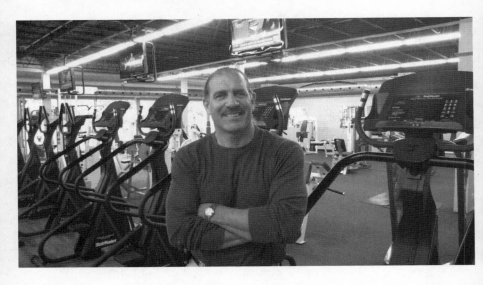

Gino A. Spada is available for hire.

With over 34 years' experience in strength training and functional training in a gym setting, this author is considered one of the elite personal trainers in Canada.

Hiring this author gives you many options. Gino can travel to you, or you can travel to him. He can do virtual assessments and consultations and design the appropriate personalized exercise program for you, or he can do all of that in person at your gym or his, as well as training you in the gym.

It is necessary to apply by way of application which is accessible by visiting www.gandmfitness.ca/training/.

Fees are à la carte and depend on the specifics of the agreement. Location of the facility, travel expenses, food and lodging if necessary, and so on will all be addressed when and if required. Fees will be quoted to successful applicants once all required information is received, reviewed, and accepted.

Printed in Canada